Medical Complications of Psychiatric Illness

Medical Complications of Psychiatric Illness

Claire Pomeroy, M.D.
James E. Mitchell, M.D.
James Roerig, Pharm.D., B.C.P.P.
Scott Crow, M.D.

American Psychiatric Publishing, Inc.
Washington, DC
London, England

Note: Each individual author has worked to ensure that all information in this book concerning drug dosages, schedules, and routes of administration is accurate as of the time of publication and consistent with standards set by the U.S. Food and Drug Administration and the general medical community. As medical research and practice advance, however, therapeutic standards may change. For this reason and because human and mechanical errors sometimes occur, it is recommended that readers follow the advice of a physician who is directly involved in their care or the care of a member of their family. A product's current package insert should be consulted for full prescribing and safety information.

Manufactured in the United States of America on acid-free paper
06 05 04 03 02 5 4 3 2 1
First Edition

American Psychiatric Publishing, Inc.
1400 K Street, N.W.
Washington, DC 20005
www.appi.org

Library of Congress Cataloging-in-Publication Data
Medical complications of psychiatric illness/Claire Pomeroy...[et al.].
p.; cm.
Includes bibliographical references and index.
ISBN 0-88048-807-7 (alk. paper)
1. Mental illness–Complications. 2. Psychology, Pathological. 3. Diagnosis, Differential. I. Pomeroy, Claire, 1955–
[DNLM: 1. Mental Disorders–diagnosis. 2. Diagnosis, Differential. 3.Diagnostic Techniques, Neurological. 4. Mental Disorders–complications. WM 141 M4887 2002]
RC454.4 .M434 2002
616.89'1–dc21

2001056175

British Library Cataloguing in Publication Data
A CIP record is available from the British Library.

Contents

Contributors

Scott Crow, M.D.
Associate Professor of Psychiatry and Director of the Eating Disorders Clinic, University of Minnesota; President, Minnesota Psychiatric Society, Minneapolis, Minnesota

James E. Mitchell, M.D.
President and Scientific Director, Neuropsychiatric Research Institute; NRI/Lee Christopherson Professor and Chair, Department of Neuroscience, University of North Dakota School of Medicine and Health Sciences, Fargo, North Dakota

Claire Pomeroy, M.D.
Professor and Chief of Infectious Disease, Department of Internal Medicine; Associate Dean for Research and Informatics; and Associate Chief of Staff, University of Kentucky College of Medicine, Lexington, Kentucky

James Roerig, Pharm.D., B.C.P.P.
Research Scientist, Neuropsychiatric Research Institute; Associate Professor of Psychiatry, Department of Neuroscience, University of North Dakota School of Medicine and Health Sciences, Fargo, North Dakota

With contributions by

Gregory Bjerke, M.D.
Staff Physician, Department of Emergency Medicine, MeritCare Health System, Fargo, North Dakota

Dean Krahn, M.D.
Chief of Psychiatry, Middleton V.A. Medical Center; Professor of Psychiatry, University of Wisconsin School of Medicine, Madison, Wisconsin

Introduction

Claire Pomeroy, M.D.
James E. Mitchell, M.D.
James Roerig, Pharm.D., B.C.P.P.
Scott Crow, M.D.

The purpose of this text is to provide practicing psychiatrists with a ready source of information concerning the medical complications of psychiatric disorders and the routine health maintenance of psychiatric patients. The authors saw these topics as ones that had been relatively neglected. Many practicing psychiatrists have deferred the general medical care of their patients to other practitioners, and in the process some have allowed their general medical skills to atrophy over time. However, there seems to be an increasing emphasis on the need for psychiatrists to assume responsibility for ensuring that their psychiatric patients receive adequate medical care. Also, there is a sizable literature suggesting that physical illness may be overlooked by psychiatrists (Felker et al. 1996; Koran et al. 1989). Hence the need for this text.

The first part of the text focuses on the general health care maintenance of these patients, including reproductive health, to aid psychiatrists in ensuring that these critical areas are addressed and that appropriate and timely referrals are made. The second part is organized by topic, focusing on those psychiatric disorders that most clearly can have medical consequences. Emphasis is placed on the use of laboratory and other diagnostic assessments.

It is important for us to point out areas that this text does not address. First, our target audience is psychiatrists who treat adult psychiatric patients rather than patients in the pediatric age group. Therefore, disorders that may have health consequences arising primarily at a young age, such as childhood autism, are not reviewed. Also, the text is not a compendium of medical illnesses that can present with psychiatric symptoms. Such reviews have been published elsewhere, and most practitioners have access to texts that summarize such information.

Our hope in writing this text is that we can provide a useful source of information for the practicing clinician and that the use of this text will contribute to improved health care for psychiatric patients, a goal we share with our readers.

REFERENCES

Felker B, Yazel JJ, Short D: Mortality and medical comorbidity among psychiatric patients: a review. Psychiatr Serv 47:1356–1363, 1996

Koran LM, Sox HC Jr, Marton KI, et al: Medical evaluation of psychiatric patients. Arch Gen Psychiatry 46:733–740, 1989

PART

I

Health Care of Psychiatric Patients

1

Routine Medical Evaluation and Health Maintenance

INTRODUCTION

Psychiatric patients have an increased rate of morbidity and mortality due to physical illnesses. Distressingly, clinicians fail to recognize these comorbid medical illnesses in nearly one-half of all cases (Brugha et al. 1989; Farmer 1987; Hankin et al. 1982; Koran et al. 1989). In a substantial percentage of patients (perhaps 10%), the physical illness is actually the cause of the psychiatric symptoms or is responsible for exacerbating the symptoms. Furthermore, the psychiatric condition itself and iatrogenic complications of medication or other treatments can result in serious medical pathology. A thorough medical evaluation should be mandatory for all new psychiatric patients (Akiskal 1994), and ongoing provision of health care should be ensured (Schwab et al. 1988).

Traditionally, many psychiatrists have been reluctant to provide the routine medical care required for psychiatric patients. An awareness of the critical interactions between somatic and mental conditions is important for the optimal care of psychiatric patients, and psychiatrists may be uniquely positioned to provide health care that bridges psychiatric and physical medicine. If psychiatrists choose not to provide these services, they should ensure that their patients have access to care from a medical physician (usually an internist or family practitioner) who is sensitive to the needs of psychiatric patients and who has expertise in their medical care. Attention to health maintenance, as well as timely treatment of acute and chronic medical conditions, will improve the health of psychiatric patients and increase the chances of successful management of their psychiatric conditions (Lima and Pai 1987).

EXCESS MORTALITY RATES IN PSYCHIATRIC PATIENTS

Psychiatric illness is clearly associated with excess mortality rates compared with the general population. Age-adjusted annual death rates from all causes among psychiatric patients are 2–4 times higher than expected (Allebeck 1989; Baxter 1996; Black and Fisher 1992; Black et al. 1985; Bruce and Leaf 1989; Crisanti and Love 1999; Curtis et al. 1996; Hannerz et al. 2001; Haugland et al. 1983; Hoyer et al. 2000; Koranyi 1977; Lawrence et al. 2000a, 2000b; Salazar-Fraile et al. 1998; Sims 1982; Sohlman and Lehtinen 1999; Tsuang and Woolson 1977; Winokur and Black 1987; Zilber et al. 1989). In a study of psychiatric outpatients, death rates during the follow-up were 1.74 times greater than expected (Martin et al. 1985a). Recent studies have suggested that standardized mortality ratios (number of deaths per year relative to the general population) in schizophrenia are 1.59 (Baxter 1996) to 2.96 (Black and Fisher 1992) to 3.34 (Mortensen and Juel 1993), depending on the study methodology used (Brown and Birthwhistle 1996). Mortality rates in major affective disorders have been reported to be 1.5 times greater than expected (Murphy et al. 1987). In one study, relative risk of death was 7 for drug addiction, 5 for alcoholism, 3 for organic disorders, 2.5 for personality disorders and neuroses, 2 for schizophrenia, and 1.5 for affective disorders compared with that of the general population (Zilber et al. 1989). In one study of patients with functional psychosis, life expectancy was reduced by one-fourth, due in particular to suicides among younger patients and cerebrovascular disease in older patients (Hannerz and Borga 2000).

Excess mortality is particularly striking soon after the diagnosis of psychosis such as schizophrenia and during or soon after psychiatric hospitalization (Hansen et al. 2001; Mortenson and Juel 1993; Simpson and Tsuang 1996). Thus, the duration of follow-up will have an impact on study findings regarding mortality in psychiatric patients.

Excess mortality rates have even been noted among patients with "pure" anxiety neurosis (Allgulander and Lavori 1991). Increased mortality is particularly noted among psychiatric patients under the age of 40 (Baxter 1996; Black and Fisher 1992; Black et al. 1985; Zilber et al. 1989). Women psychiatric patients may be at higher relative risk than men (Baxter 1996; Black and Fisher 1992). In past decades, the increased risk of premature death was even higher than it is currently (Babigian and Odoroff 1969; Rorsman 1974).

Causes of death for psychiatric patients include those directly attributable to the psychiatric disorder as well as "natural" causes. Not unexpectedly, suicide and accidents are reported as the main causes for excess mortality rates in this population (Winokur and Black 1987; Zilber et al. 1989). Although some controversy exists regarding whether increased rates of premature deaths due to natural causes still occur today (Black et al. 1985; Eastwood 1975; Martin et al. 1985b), most studies suggest that greater risk persists for death due to certain medical problems (Simpson and Tsuang 1996; Winokur and Black 1987; Zilber et al. 1989). The identification of specific causes of excess death among psychiatric patients has been the focus of many studies. Increased death rates due to infectious and respiratory conditions are reported most frequently (Allebeck 1989; Black et al. 1985; Mortensen and Juel 1993; Saugstad and Odegard 1979), especially among institutionalized patients (Zilber et al. 1989) and in persons with schizophrenia (Tsuang et al. 1980). Among psychiatric patients, death rates for cardiovascular disease have been reported to be both higher (Mortensen and Juel 1993; Penninx et al. 2001) and lower (Zilber et al. 1989) than in the general population. Variable results have been obtained for studies of death rates from cancer—suggesting that rates may be higher (Black et al. 1985; Zilber et al. 1989), lower (Murphy et al. 1987; Shekelle et al. 1981), or the same as in the general population (Modrzewska and Book 1979). One study suggested that cancer mortality is higher in psychiatric patients, even though cancer incidence is comparable with that of the general population (Lawrence et al. 2000a).

MEDICAL MORBIDITY IN PSYCHIATRIC PATIENTS

Medical comorbidity is well documented in psychiatric patients. Unfortunately, medical illnesses often remain unrecognized or untreated in this patient population (Barnes et al. 1983; Burke 1972, 1978; Davies 1965; Forsythe et al. 1977; Hall et al. 1980; Koranyi 1972; Moos and Mertens 1996; Muecke and Krueger 1981; Tsuang et al. 1983; Wells et al. 1989).

Diagnosed psychiatric illnesses may actually represent unrecognized physical illnesses (Warnes 1982). A wide variety of physical illnesses can present with predominantly psychiatric symptoms (Table 1–1).

Studies have reported that patients with physical illness misdiagnosed as psychiatric disease represent 6% (Koran et al. 1989), 9.1% (Hall et al. 1978, 1981), 18.7% (Summers et al. 1981), and 20% (Koranyi 1979) of psychiatric patients.

Traditionally, neurosyphilis was responsible for a large portion of psychiatric admissions (Dewhurst 1969). Metabolic illnesses including porphyria (Tishler et al. 1985); vitamin deficiencies; endocrine disorders such as untreated thyroid disease; neurological diseases including degenerative diseases, vasculitides, seizures, and tumors; and a variety of other

Table 1–1. Physical illnesses or conditions that can present as psychiatric diagnoses

Metabolic
- Acute intermittent porphyria
- Nutritional deficiency, especially thiamine, B_6, B_{12}, niacin, folate
- Pheochromocytoma or carcinoid

Endocrine
- Thyroid abnormalities
- Cushing's or Addison's disease
- Diabetes mellitus
- Parathyroid disorders
- Hyper- or hypocalcemia, hyper- or hypophosphatemia, hyper- or hypomagnesemia
- Hypoglycemia
- Pernicious anemia

Rheumatologic
- Systemic lupus erythematosus
- Other vasculitides

Cardiovascular
- Angina, arrythmias
- Hypertension

Pulmonary
- Hypoxia
- Pulmonary emboli

Iatrogenic
- Medication side effects

Renal
- Uremia

Infectious
- Central nervous system infections, encephalitis
- Malaria, other systemic infections

Neurologic
- Seizure disorders, especially temporal lobe epilepsy
- Brain abscess
- Neurosyphilis
- "Slow virus" diseases, e.g., Creutzfeldt-Jakob, subacute sclerosing panencephalitis
- Brain tumors (glioma, meningioma), cerebrovascular accidents, subdural hematoma, and other central nervous system lesions
- Alzheimer's/dementia/delirium
- Multiple sclerosis
- Degenerative central nervous system diseases, e.g., Huntington's chorea

Gastrointestinal
- Hepatitis/other causes of hepatic failure
- Wilson's disease
- Gastrointestinal abnormalities presenting as eating disorders

Other
- Menopause
- Cancers—multiple types, especially if advanced or with paraneoplastic syndrome
- Heavy metal poisoning
- Drug abuse or withdrawal
- Alcohol abuse or withdrawal

medical illnesses can masquerade as primary psychiatric disorders. Tragically, if appropriate medical evaluation is overlooked (Koranyi 1979), critical delays in therapy may result in patient deaths or disability. Although heightened awareness and the wider availability of laboratory testing have likely decreased the frequency of misdiagnosis, psychiatrists and other health care providers must remain vigilant in ruling out physical illness as a cause of apparent psychiatric symptoms.

Of equal import are the many physical illnesses that complicate or coexist with psychiatric illnesses (Table 1–2).

Table 1–2. Medical complications of psychiatric illnesses

Increased mortality rates Due to events attributable to psychiatric illnesses (i.e., suicide, accidents) Due to "natural" causes	**Gastrointestinal** Altered gastrointestinal function (often due to medications) Alcoholic liver disease
Cardiovascular Increased rates of atherosclerosis (?—Increased incidence of hypertension)	**Neurological** Increased incidence of neurologic abnormalities
Endocrine Increased incidence of diabetes mellitus (?—secondary to medications) Polyuria, polydipsia (secondary to antipsychotics)	**Renal** Hyponatremia secondary to polyuria
Genitourinary Increased infection risk (?—due to poor hygiene, institutionalization)	**Immunologic** Altered immune system function
Rheumatologic Variable reports of impact on arthritis	**Nutritional** Poor diet Vitamin deficiencies
Dermatologic Ulcers, skin breakdown (due to lifestyle, institutionalization)	**Substance abuse** Increased likelihood of cigarette use Increased likelihood of alcohol use Increased illicit substance abuse
Respiratory Increase in chronic lung disease (?—due to cigarette use) Increase in pneumonia (?—due to institutionalization)	**Other** (?—Altered incidence of cancer) Increased pain tolerance Lack of exercise High-risk sexual behaviors
	Iatrogenic Medication side effects

One-third to one-half of psychiatric patients have identifiable physical illness (Bunce et al. 1982; Burke 1972, 1978; Dalmau et al. 1998; Felker et al. 1996; Schiffer et al. 1988; Summers et al. 1981). In the classic report by Koranyi (1979), 43% of psychiatric clinic patients had at least one physical illness, and in nearly one-half of the cases, the physical illness was unrecognized by the referring health care provider. In a later study, 80% of patients admitted to a state psychiatric hospital had physical illnesses requiring treatment, including 46% in whom the medical illness was unrecognized and had caused or exacerbated the psychiatric illness (Hall et al. 1981). In another study, 41.3% of psychiatric patients had a physical medical problem, and 65% of the diagnoses were previously unsuspected (Summers et al. 1981). These findings are consistent with another report in which 45% of psychiatric patients had an active, significant physical disease, with only 47% of these recognized by the mental health care providers. Active physical disease was significantly more common in state hospital patients (57%) than in day-treatment patients (28%) or patients living in nursing facilities (25%) (Koran et al. 1989).

For elderly psychiatric patients, the risk of concomitant physical illness is even more significant (Gierz and Jeste 1993; Lacro and Jeste 1994). Elderly psychiatric inpatients suffered from a mean of 5.6 active medical problems in one study (Zubenko et al. 1997). In another study, 92% of geriatric psychiatric inpatients had at least one diagnosable significant medical problem (Sheline 1990).

Cardiovascular disease appears to be the most prevalent somatic disease in psychiatric patients, followed by central nervous system abnormalities, endocrine disturbances, nutritional problems, metabolic illnesses, and infections (Bunce et al. 1982; Hall et al. 1981). In a study of the prevalence of physical illnesses in geriatric psychiatric inpatients, cardiovascular disease was most prevalent (34%), followed by neurological (22%), genitourinary (17%), respiratory (17%), and gastrointestinal (17%) disorders (Sheline 1990). In another study, genitourinary problems were most frequent (22%), with cardiovascular (15%), blood and connective tissue (11%), respiratory (11%), skin (11%), and metabolic problems (8%) also frequently found.

Lifetime prevalences of chronic lung disease, heart disease, hypertension, arthritis, and neurological diseases have been reported to be significantly greater in patients with an affective disorder than in the general population (Wells et al. 1989). An increased risk of cardiovascular illnesses has been reported in psychiatric patients (Baldwin 1979; Bunce et al. 1982), especially in patients with affective disorders (Harris 1988); the findings are less clear in schizophrenia. Traditionally, the incidence of infectious diseases, especially tuberculosis and pneumonias, was exceedingly high among psychiatric patients (Baldwin 1979). Although this excess risk has lessened somewhat in the era of deinstitutionalization, an increased frequency of infectious diseases persists.

Reasons for the apparent increased risk of diabetes among patients with schizophrenia remain incompletely defined. The frequency with which diabetes mellitus is overlooked in psychiatric patients has been emphasized (Koranyi 1979). Glucose metabolism is often abnormal in patients with schizophrenia (Brambilla et al. 1976). Various mechanisms have been postulated, including medication side effects as well as inherent biological susceptibility. The known tendency of neuroleptics to induce glucose intolerance may contribute.

Conversely, a reduced incidence of asthma, hay fever, and other allergic phenomena has been reported in patients with schizophrenia

(Baldwin 1979). Several studies have reported a negative association between rheumatoid arthritis and schizophrenia (Eaton et al. 1992; Harris 1988), although the pathogenesis remains elusive. A negative relationship between cancer and schizophrenia has been proposed but is controversial due to conflicting study results (Baldwin 1979; Jeste et al. 1996).

A variety of neurological abnormalities have been described in psychiatric patients, especially those with schizophrenia (Torrey 1980; Woods et al. 1986). These are usually soft neurological signs, and specific therapeutic interventions are rarely indicated. Neurological soft signs have also been reported in patients with mania (Mukherjee et al. 1984; Nasrallah et al. 1983). Some of these abnormalities may be due to prolonged treatment with neuroleptics, but a common biological propensity has also been postulated.

Other psychiatric disorders appear to be associated with increased risk for physical illnesses. For example, medical disorders that may mimic, precipitate, or complicate panic disorder include thyroid disease, pheochromocytoma, hypoglycemia, temporal lobe epilepsy, and possibly mitral valve prolapse (Stein 1986).

Psychiatric illness can also interfere with the management of and recovery from physical illness. The negative impact of depression on recovery from myocardial infarction (Connerney et al. 2001; Frasure-Smith et al. 1993; Schleifer et al. 1989), congestive heart failure (Jiang et al. 2001), stroke (Parikh et al. 1990), chronic obstructive pulmonary disease (Weaver and Narsavage 1992), arthritis (Beckham et al. 1992), Parkinson's disease (Starkstein and Robinson 1989), and medical illness requiring hospitalization (von Ammon Cavanaugh et al. 2001) is well documented. This problem has been particularly noted among older patients (Katz et al. 1994). Comorbid psychiatric conditions have been shown to increase the number of hospital admissions needed and the length of stay (Saravay et al. 1991; Savoca 1999).

REASONS FOR EXCESS MORBIDITY AND MORTALITY IN PSYCHIATRIC PATIENTS

The reasons for the excess morbidity and mortality due to somatic illness observed in psychiatric patients remain incompletely defined. Both biological and social reasons have been proposed (Cohen and Rodriguez 1995; Sims 1987) (Table 1–3).

It has been hypothesized that patients with schizophrenia and possibly other psychiatric patients possess an inherent biological predisposition that might lead to an increased risk of somatic disease and death

Table 1–3. Postulated reasons for increased medical morbidity and mortality rates in psychiatric patients

Biological

Suicide, self-injury

Genetic cosusceptibility to psychiatric and physical illness

Adverse impact of psychiatric condition on physical condition, e.g., stress causing immune dysfunction

Poor health maintenance

- Substance abuse—alcohol, cigarettes, illicit drugs
- Other impaired health-related behaviors—e.g., poor diet, lack of exercise

Pain tolerance and other sensory deficits

Poor compliance with medication or other health care recommendations

Medication side effects

Risks of institutionalization

- Overcrowding
- Inadequate diet
- Lack of exercise

Social

Poor socioeconomic conditions leading to higher-risk lifestyle

- Poor housing
- Lack of education
- Inadequate clothing
- Interaction with other disenfranchised populations

Lack of access to health care for established medical illnesses

- Poor finances
- Lack of transportation
- Lack of patient knowledge of available resources

Lack of access to preventative health care

Interference of illness with social skills needed to access health care

- Symptoms obscure historical clues
- Patient unable to recognize or communicate accurate history
- Symptoms interfere with ability to cooperate with physical examination
- Symptoms preclude adequate diagnostic tests or therapeutic intervention

Failure of health care workers to recognize physical illness in psychiatric patients

Health care provider prejudice, leading to suboptimal medical care

(Kendell 1975). A variety of factors attributable to treatment of the psychiatric illness, especially medications and institutionalization, can also cause physical problems. In addition, myriad social forces can cause medical complications in the psychiatric patient or prevent access to treatment for medical illnesses, thus markedly increasing the risk of disease chronicity or death.

The most obvious causes of increased morbidity and mortality in psychiatric patients are events directly attributable to the psychiatric illness. Suicide is far and away the most important cause of death in psychiatric patients, contributing to excess mortality in affective disorders, schizophrenia, and many other psychiatric illnesses. Other medical complications directly related to the psychiatric problem can also contribute to death, such as inanition in persons with anorexia nervosa, electrolyte disturbances in individuals with bulimia nervosa, drug overdose in addicted individuals, cirrhosis in alcoholic individuals, polydipsia in persons with schizophrenia, and trauma in patients with self-injurious behaviors (de Leon et al. 1994 and as reviewed throughout this book).

The adverse consequences of medications and other psychiatric treatments, including psychosurgery, restraints, and electroconvulsive therapy, may be responsible for some of the increased risk of morbidity and death among psychiatric patients. Neuroleptic medications may cause medical morbidity, including tardive dyskinesia and glucose intolerance. Furthermore, some psychiatric medications, such as the phenothiazines, tricyclic antidepressants, and anxiolytics, may increase pain thresholds and potentially delay recognition of serious intercurrent medical illnesses.

Institutionalization is well recognized as a cause of increased somatic morbidity and mortality among psychiatric patients. Traditionally, patients in psychiatric institutions commonly were exposed to major outbreaks of infectious illnesses caused by overcrowding, poor hygiene, substandard physical facilities, and poor infection control. As the use of institutionalization for psychiatric illnesses has decreased and the quality of facilities has increased, this has become less of a problem. Nevertheless, rates of infections such as tuberculosis, hepatitis, and communicable respiratory and gastrointestinal infections among institutionalized individuals far exceed those of the general population and place these patients at risk of short- and long-term medical complications.

Cosusceptibility to psychiatric and physical illnesses has been postulated. Clearly, understanding of the interactions between the brain and the rest of the body has advanced in recent years, as evidenced by the emerging field of psychoneuroimmunology. The adverse effect of psychiatric illness on physical condition has now been amply demonstrated for various disease processes. The association of depression and stress with immune dysfunction (Maes et al. 1991), potentially leading to increased risk of infection or malignancies, has been documented. It has been suggested that the platelet response to activation in patients with major depression is supersensitive, possibly explaining the increased risk of cardiovascular mortality in this patient population (Berk and Plein

2000). It also has been hypothesized that polydipsia, atypical responses to medications, and high rates of tobacco consumption are manifestations of genes linked to schizophrenia (Josiassen and Schindler 1996).

Poor health maintenance behaviors characterize many psychiatric populations and undoubtedly are responsible for many of the physical illnesses that affect patients with mental illness. Patients with schizophrenia and other psychiatric patients have higher-than-average rates of alcohol abuse, illicit drug use, cigarette smoking, and caffeine consumption (Jeste et al. 1996; Mueser et al. 1992; Regier et al. 1990). High frequency of cigarette use by these patients (Glassman 1993) places them at increased risk of pulmonary disease (Mortensen and Juel 1993). Alcohol is used in excess by many patients, often to self-medicate their psychiatric symptoms. Cocaine and other illicit stimulant drugs are abused more frequently by persons with schizophrenia and other patients with psychiatric illnesses than by the general population (Brady et al. 1990). Medical complications of such abuse markedly increase the rates of morbidity and mortality. Other poor health maintenance behaviors less directly but no less assuredly increase rates of physical disease and death among psychiatric patients. Poor diet, lack of exercise, inadequate clothing, suboptimal housing, and lack of education have all been associated with increased physical morbidity and mortality. Furthermore, patients with psychiatric illnesses are less likely to be married—a risk factor for premature death (Johnson et al. 2000). Finally, psychiatrically ill patients are often poor and as a result may tend to lead a higher-risk lifestyle. Interactions with other disenfranchised populations place these patients at increased risk of injury, communicable diseases, and even death.

In some psychiatric patients, biological or genetic factors may be present that explain increased rates of physical illness. For example, it has been proposed that individuals with schizophrenia have higher pain thresholds (Dworkin 1994) and other sensory deficits that may cause them to minimize physical symptoms and further decrease their likelihood of accessing needed health care. It has been suggested that anosognosia (i.e. ignorance, real or feigned, of the presence of disease) contributes to the high rates of medical comorbidity in patients with schizophrenia (Jeste et al. 1996). Many psychotic patients are unwilling or unable to communicate discomfort or pain, even in the face of life-threatening illnesses (Kampmeier 1977; Talbott and Linn 1978). Sensory impairments, including visual or hearing loss or distortion, have been reported in schizophrenia and mood disorders, especially among older patients and in patients with a late onset of their psychiatric illness (Prager and Jeste 1993), and may contribute to inability to sense symptoms of physical illness.

As important as these biological explanations for increased risk of somatic illness in psychiatric patients are, social explanations are often even more significant. Lack of understanding or motivation may prevent the psychiatric patient from complying with health care worker recommendations, thus increasing the risk of disease progression, misdiagnosis, or failure to procure adequate therapies. Lack of access to health care is a major cause of increased morbidity and mortality rates among psychiatric patients (Berren et al. 1999; Jeste et al. 1996). Poverty, homelessness, lack of insurance, lack of transportation, and lack of education may all directly prevent the psychiatric patient from receiving adequate health care. Although these issues must be addressed through larger social change, psychiatrists must be cognizant of their impact on the psychiatric patient's ability to obtain needed medical services.

Equally disturbing, health care workers may fail to accurately diagnose or manage medical illnesses in the psychiatric patient. Psychiatric symptoms may obscure the physical symptoms or prevent the patient from adequately reporting symptoms and other historical information to the provider. In one study, 70% of psychiatric inpatients were assessed to be unable to communicate adequately with their physician (Bunce et al. 1982). This may be due to health care provider prejudice, failure to train health care workers to recognize physical illness in psychiatric patients, or time constraints that make it difficult for many clinicians to spend the amount of time necessary to adequately assess the medical needs of these persons. Furthermore, psychiatrically ill patients may invoke negative feelings in the physician. As a result, medical evaluation of psychiatric patients is often cursory or omitted altogether. Regardless of the cause, lack of adequate preventative services as well as lack of appropriate and timely treatment of acute and chronic medical problems is a major determinant of increased physical disease rates among psychiatric patients.

ROLE OF THE PSYCHIATRIST

Despite the high prevalence of medical illness in psychiatric patients, thorough medical evaluation of psychiatric patients often does not occur and/or is not available in either psychiatric or other medical settings (Bunce et al. 1982). The compartmentalization of medical education and subsequent specialty training has resulted in the lack of a comprehensive patient care approach that considers both the somatic and psychological problems of the patient (Leeman 1975). Unique challenges are posed by the psychiatric patient. As a result, medically ill psychiatric patients are too often rejected from medical clinics or hospitals and transferred to forensic or psychiatric facilities where correct diagnosis and treatment of medical problems may be overlooked (Bunce et al. 1982).

Clearly, many psychiatrists do not believe that medical evaluation for physical illness is within the purview of their practice. In one survey, fewer than 35% of practicing psychiatrists routinely physically examined their patients, and 32% of the psychiatrists indicated that they did not feel competent to perform a physical examination (McIntyre and Romano 1977). In another survey of psychiatrists, none of the respondents routinely performed physical examinations on new outpatients, and most psychiatrists with inpatient practices delegated the hospital admission physical examination to other physicians (Patterson 1978). Fifty-three percent of the respondents indicated that they did not perform physical examinations because they no longer felt competent to do so. Others avoided examining patients to prevent transference and countertransference problems. Some psychiatrists admitted that they just did not like performing physical examinations (Patterson 1978). The validity of concerns about negative transference precipitated by physical examinations is controversial (Busch and Cavanaugh 1985; Summers and Munoz 1981), and examples of positive psychological outcomes of performing a physical examination have been reported (Schiffer et al. 1988).

The risks of the psychiatrist depending on a medical "clearance" by the patient's family doctor, internist, pediatrician, or gynecologist have been emphasized (Sternberg 1986). Studies reveal that simple referral of the psychiatric patient to other physicians for examination of possible physical illness frequently proves insufficient (Sternberg 1986). Thus, if psychiatrists choose not to perform physical examinations or manage medical complications, it is crucial that they identify medical practitioners with particular expertise in caring for psychiatric patients to perform this function (Berren et al. 1999). Then, ongoing dialogue between the psychiatrist and the medical physician must be prioritized to optimize patient care (Druss and Rosenheck 1997).

INITIAL MEDICAL EVALUATION

Many medical care systems fail to ensure that physical diseases will be diagnosed and treated on the patient's arrival within a psychiatric setting (Felker et al. 1996; Moos and Mertens 1996). As mentioned previously, reliance on the notion of "medical clearance" of the psychiatric patient by other physicians is not adequate unless the extent of the referring physician's evaluation is known (Schiffer et al. 1988). New managed care requirements and shrinking reimbursement may further exacerbate the risk of incomplete, cursory medical examinations. Psychiatrists who elect not to perform these functions should assume responsibility for reviewing the results of the medical evaluation, assessing thoroughness, and determining if further work-up or referral is needed.

The optimal content of the initial medical evaluation remains to be defined. Some authors have recommended an extensive diagnostic battery for all new psychiatric patients, especially those being hospitalized, to include routine physical, psychiatric, and neurologic examinations, complete blood count, screening renal and liver function tests, urinalysis, electrocardiogram, and sleep-deprived electroencephalogram (Hall et al. 1980). Others have emphasized that a complete history and physical examination with directed laboratory evaluation is appropriate and more cost-effective (Roca et al. 1987). Methodologies for a psychiatric physical examination (Schiffer et al. 1988; Summers and Munoz 1981) have been described in detail, as have suggestions for a more detailed neurologic examination (Granacher 1981; Schiffer et al. 1988).

Some authors have proposed routine medical evaluations tailored to specific psychiatric conditions. For example, Stein (1986) recommends a routine panic disorder workup to rule out underlying medical causes of the psychiatric symptoms. Specifically, the suggested evaluation includes a general medical history; family history; general physical examination with attention to the thyroid gland, blood pressure, and the cardiac system; and laboratory evaluation with a complete blood count, serum electrolytes, calcium and phosphorus measurements, urinalysis, and thyroid function tests, but not routine evaluation for pheochromocytoma or hypoglycemia.

Appropriate use of the laboratory in psychiatry has been the focus of many reports (Martin and Preskorn 1986). For example, laboratory studies for evaluation of dementia may include complete blood count, syphilis serologies, metabolic screenings, thyroid function tests, serum folate and B_{12} levels, urinalysis, chest X ray, and head computed tomography scans (Martin and Preskorn 1986; Thomas 1979). Drug screens may be needed for patients with acute psychosis, panic disorder, or anxiety. Thyroid function tests have yielded abnormal results in a significant portion of newly admitted psychiatric patients (Cohen and Swigar 1979). The laboratory plays a critical role in appropriate monitoring of psychotropic drug levels (Martin and Preskorn 1986).

Routine use of head computed tomography or magnetic resonance imaging scans has been shown not to be cost-effective for psychiatric patients. Use of such scans should probably be restricted to evaluation of patients with focal neurologic findings or historical clues such as head trauma or sudden onset of symptoms that suggest the possibility of structural intracranial abnormalities (Larson et al. 1981). The use of other visual imaging techniques is generally limited to research at this time. For example, tests have indicated frontal hypoactivity in schizophrenia, as evidenced by decreased blood flow by regional cerebral blood flow studies and decreased glucose utilization by positron emission tomography studies (Martin and Preskorn 1986).

PURPOSE OF THE HEALTH MAINTENANCE VISIT

Because psychiatrists are often the only physicians consulted by chronic psychiatric outpatients, they can play an important role in the ongoing medical care of these patients (Table 1–4).

Ideally, the psychiatrist will be sensitive to possible medical problems, investigate physical complaints when they arise, refer to consultants when appropriate, and coordinate psychiatric and medical treatment on a continuing basis (Barnes et al. 1983). The psychiatrist may be uniquely able to assess for possible medication side effects, because many primary care providers are not as aware of the myriad complications potentially associated with these drugs. Furthermore, it has been suggested that for this population the psychiatrist should be willing to assume many of the functions typically associated with the primary care physician (Fink 1977; Oken and Fink 1976). Alternatively, the psychiatrist should ensure that patients are being seen by a primary care provider and should communicate with that physician on a regular basis.

Table 1–4. Purposes of health maintenance visit for psychiatric patients

Evaluate for medical causes of psychiatric symptoms
Monitor for medical complications of psychiatric illness
Monitor for adverse medical consequences of therapies for psychiatric illness, especially drug side effects
Routine health maintenance
Early detection of medical illnesses
Prevention of medical illnesses
Optimize lifestyle to achieve "wellness"

RECOMMENDATIONS FOR THE HEALTH MAINTENANCE VISIT

Psychiatric diagnoses do not preclude the need for preventative health services and, as outlined above, may actually increase the need for such medical care. Consensus recommendations for health maintenance visits are now available from the American College of Physicians (Eddy 1991), the Canadian Task Force on the Periodic Health Examination (1987), and the U.S. Preventative Services Task Force (1989) and have been well summarized (Friedman 1992; Hayward et al. 1991; Kern and Roberts 1995; Kligman and Hale 1994; Sox 1994).

The cornerstone of the health maintenance visit is the history and physical examination (Table 1–5).

After the initial visit, an interim history and physical examination that focuses on areas related to medical problems for which the patient is at risk should be performed (Hayward et al. 1991). All patients should have blood pressure monitored at least every 2 years. For women, annual breast examinations after age 40, with the use of mammography beginning at age 50 (and possibly at age 40), are recommended. Cervical cytologic screening (Pap smear) is indicated every 1–3 years. Further information is available in Chapter 2.

Most routine screening laboratory tests have generally been shown not to be cost-effective. Serum cholesterol measurement every 5 years in adults has been recommended. Other laboratory evaluation is not routinely advised but should be directed at evaluation of any medical problems suggested by the history and physical examination or for which patients are at high risk by virtue of their family history, lifestyle, or medical therapies.

One of the most cost-effective interventions is vaccination. For adults, it should be ascertained that all appropriate childhood vaccinations were received. Tetanus booster vaccine should be administered every 10 years. After age 65, yearly influenza vaccinations and provision of pneumococcal vaccine (once and possibly repeated after 10 years) are required. Patients in risk groups should receive additional vaccines, such as hepatitis B immunization or vaccines required for travel.

Physician counseling regarding healthy lifestyles is an integral part of the health maintenance visit and can be effective. Counseling regarding the risks of cigarette smoking (Thorndike et al. 2001), excess alcohol use, and illicit drugs is the responsibility of every physician. Recommendations about seat belt use and the importance of exercise and a healthful diet are also essential components of good health care. Health care

Table 1–5. Recommended components of the health maintenance visit

History
- Interval medical history
- Diet/exercise pattern
- Tobacco/alcohol/drug use
- Injury prevention practices
- Sexual practices, including assessment of risk for HIV/sexually transmitted diseases

Physical examination
- Vital signs—height, weight, blood pressure, pulse
- Oral cavity examination, including dental
- Screening examination of major organ systems
- Breast and pelvic examination (women)
- Testicular examination (men)
- Rectal examination
- Visual/hearing screening

Functional assessment
- Living situation
- Employment
- Family/friends support network
- Need for community support agency referrals

Screening laboratory evaluations
- Cholesterol
- Stool for occult blood
- Others as guided by history/physical

Screening diagnostic tests
- Pap smear (women)
- Mammogram (women ages 40–50 and older)
- Others as guided by history and/or physical examination

Immunizations
- Tetanus/diphtheria booster (every 10 years)
- Influenza (annually if elderly/high risk)
- MMR, hepatitis B, pneumococcal vaccine (when indicated)

Counseling
- Diet recommendations
- Exercise regimens
- Prevention of tobacco/alcohol/illicit drug use
- Sexual practices including safe sex and contraceptive advice
- Breast (women)/testicular (men) self-examination

Other
- Monitoring based on potential complications of psychiatric illness and treatment (tailored to the individual patient)

Note. See text for recommended frequency of each component and further details. MMR = measles, mumps, and rubella vaccine.

workers should assess the sexual practices of their patients. High rates of sexually transmitted diseases including HIV are a major problem in our society today, and counseling about safe sex practices and contraceptive techniques is critical. Some authors have advocated developing a series of mini-counseling sessions (3–10 minutes in length) (Kligman and Hale 1994), and others have pointed out the benefit of written patient education materials (Kern and Roberts 1995), especially handouts to send home with the patient for review.

Psychiatrists may elect to perform some or all of the components of the health maintenance visit themselves or to defer some portions to the primary care provider or physician extender. Although preventive care is often overlooked because of limited time, inadequate resources, or inexperience, it is now recognized that these practices are cost-effective. Nevertheless, psychiatrists should be aware that truncated appointment times, limited access, and bureaucratic requirements entailed by changing reimbursement requirements may interfere with the patient's ability to access these services. Psychiatrists can improve their patients' overall health by ensuring that they are not denied the benefits of routine preventative care.

SUMMARY

Many medical illnesses can complicate psychiatric illness. In addition, physical illness can be misdiagnosed as psychiatric in origin. Therefore, psychiatrists must be cognizant of potential medical complications in their patients. It is each psychiatrist's responsibility to either assume primary medical care responsibility or ensure that an expert consulting medical physician is involved in the patient's care. In the latter case, ongoing dialogue between the psychiatrist and the primary care provider is mandatory. Awareness of the health maintenance needs of psychiatric patients is an important first step toward reducing the increased mortality and morbidity rates observed in patients with psychiatric illnesses, thus optimizing the health of these patients.

REFERENCES

Akiskal HS: The mental status examination, in The Medical Basis of Psychiatry. Edited by Winokur G, Clayton P. Philadelphia, PA, WB Saunders, 1994, pp 3–15

Allebeck P: Schizophrenia: a life-shortening disease. Schizophr Bull 15:81–89, 1989

Allgulander C, Lavori PW: Excess mortality among 3302 patients with "pure" anxiety neurosis. Arch Gen Psychiatry 48:599–602, 1991

Babigian HM, Odoroff CL: The mortality experience of a population with psychiatric disease. Am J Psychiatry 126:52–62, 1969

Baldwin JA: Schizophrenia and physical disease. Psychol Med 6:611–618, 1979

Barnes RF, Mason JC, Greer C, et al: Medical illness in chronic psychiatric outpatients. Gen Hosp Psychiatry 5:191–195, 1983

Baxter DN: The mortality experience of individuals on the Salford psychiatric case register, I: all case mortality. Br J Psychiatry 168:772–779, 1996

Beckham JC, D'Amico CJ, Rice R, et al: Depression and level of functioning in patients with rheumatoid arthritis. Can J Psychiatry 37:539–543, 1992

Berk M, Plein H: Platelet supersensitivity to thrombin stimulation in depression: a possible mechanism for the association with cardiovascular mortality. Clin Neuropharmacol 23:182–185, 2000

Berren MR, Santiago JM, Zent MR, et al: Health care utilization by persons with severe and persistent mental illness. Psychiatr Serv 50:559–561, 1999

Black DW, Fisher R: Mortality of DSM-III-R schizophrenia. Schizophr Res 7:109–116, 1992

Black DW, Warrack G, Winokur G: Excess mortality among psychiatric patients. JAMA 253:58–61, 1985

Brady KT, Anton R, Ballenger JC, et al: Cocaine abuse among schizophrenic patients. Am J Psychiatry 147:1164–1167, 1990

Brambilla F, Guastalla A, Guerrini A, et al: Glucose-insulin metabolism in chronic schizophrenia. Diseases of the Nervous System 37:98–103, 1976

Brown AS, Birthwhistle J: Excess mortality of mental illness. Br J Psychiatry 169:383–384, 1996

Bruce ML, Leaf PJ: Psychiatric disorders and 15-month mortality in a community sample of older adults. Am J Public Health 79:727–730, 1989

Brugha TS, Wing JK, Smith BL: Physical health of the long-term mentally ill in the community: is there unmet need? Br J Psychiatry 155:777–781, 1989

Bunce DF II, Jones LR, Badger LW, et al: Medical illness in psychiatric patients: barriers to diagnosis and treatment. South Med J 75:941–944, 1982

Burke AW: Physical illness in psychiatric hospital patients in Jamaica. Br J Psychiatry 121:321–322, 1972

Burke AW: Physical disorder among day hospital patients. Br J Psychiatry 133:22–27, 1978

Busch KA, Cavanaugh JL: Physical examination of psychiatric patients: medical and legal issues. Hosp Community Psychiatry 36:958–961, 1985

Canadian Task Force on the Periodic Health Examination: The periodic health examination, 2. Can Med Assoc J 138:618–626, 1987

Cohen KL, Swigar ME: Thyroid function screening in psychiatric patients. JAMA 242:254–257, 1979

Cohen S, Rodriguez MS: Pathways linking affective disturbance and physical disorders. Health Psychol 14:374–380, 1995

Connerney I, Shapiro PA, McLaughlin JS, et al: Relation between depression after coronary artery bypass surgery and 12-month outcome: a prospective study. Lancet 358:1766–1771, 2001

Crisanti AS, Love EJ: Mortality among involuntarily admitted psychiatric patients: a survival analysis. Soc Psychiatry Psychiatr Epidemiol 34:627–633, 1999

Curtis JL, Millman EJ, Struening E, et al: Deaths among former psychiatric inpatients in an outreach case management program. Psychiatr Serv 47:398–402, 1996

Dalmau AB, Bergman BK, Brismar BG: Somatic morbidity among patients diagnosed with affective psychoses and paranoid disorders. Psychosomatics 39:253–262, 1998

Davies DW: Physical illness in psychiatric out-patients. Br J Psychiatry 111:27–33, 1965

de Leon J, Verghese C, Tracy JI, et al: Polydipsia and water intoxication in psychiatric patients: a review of the epidemiological literature. Biol Psychiatry 35:408–419, 1994

Dewhurst K: The neurosyphilitic psychoses today: a survey of 91 patients. Br J Psychiatry 115:31–38, 1969

Druss BG, Rosenheck RA: Use of medical services by veterans with mental disorders. Psychosomatics 38:451–458, 1997

Dworkin RH: Pain insensitivity in schizophrenia: a neglected phenomenon and some implications. Schizophr Bull 20:235–248, 1994

Eastwood MR: The Relationship Between Physical and Mental Illness. Toronto, Canada, University of Toronto Press, 1975

Eaton WW, Hayward C, Ram R: Schizophrenia and rheumatoid arthritis: a review. Schizophr Rev 6:181–192, 1992

Eddy DM: Common Screening Tests. Philadelphia, PA, American College of Physicians, 1991

Farmer S: Medical problems of chronic patients in a community support program. Hosp Community Psychiatry 38:745–749, 1987

Felker B, Yazel JJ, Short D: Mortality and medical comorbidity among psychiatric patients: a review. Psychiatr Serv 47:1356–1363, 1996

Fink PJ: The relationship of psychiatry to primary care. Am J Psychiatry 134:126–129, 1977

Forsythe RJ, Ilk CR, Bard J, et al: Primary medical care in psychiatry. Curr Psychiatr Ther 17:91–97, 1977

Frasure-Smith N, Lesperance F, Talajic M: Depression following myocardial infarction: impact on 6-month survival. JAMA 270:1819–1825, 1993

Friedman GD: The preventative health examination, in Cecil's Textbook of Medicine. Edited by Wyngaarden JB, Smith LH, Bennett JC. Philadelphia, PA, WB Saunders, 1992, pp 61–62

Gierz M, Jeste DV: Physical comorbidity in elderly schizophrenic and depressed patients. Am J Geriatr Psychiatry 1:165–170, 1993

Glassman AH: Cigarette smoking: implications for psychiatric illness. Am J Psychiatry 150:546–553, 1993

Granacher RP: The neurologic examination in geriatric psychiatry. Psychosomatics 22:485–499, 1981

Hall RCW, Popkin MK, Devaul RA, et al: Physical illness presenting as psychiatric illness. Arch Gen Psychiatry 35:1315–1320, 1978

Hall RCW, Gardner ER, Stickney SK, et al: Physical illness manifesting as psychiatric disease, II: analysis of a state hospital inpatient population. Arch Gen Psychiatry 37:989–995, 1980

Hall RCW, Gardner ER, Popkin MK, et al: Unrecognized physical illness prompting psychiatric admission: a prospective study. Am J Psychiatry 138:629–635, 1981

Hankin JR, Steinwachs DM, Regier DA, et al: Use of general medical care services by persons with mental disorders. Arch Gen Psychiatry 39:225–231, 1982

Hannerz H, Borga P: Mortality among persons with a history as psychiatric inpatients with functional psychosis. Soc Psychiatry Psychiatr Epidemiol 35:380–387, 2000

Hannerz H, Borga P, Borritz M: Life expectancies for individuals with psychiatric diagnoses. Public Health 115:328–337, 2001

Hansen V, Jacobsen BK, Arnesen E: Cause-specific mortality in psychiatric patients after deinstitutionalisation. Br J Psychiatry 179:438–443, 2001

Harris AE: Physical disease and schizophrenia. Schizophr Bull 14:85–96, 1988

Haugland G, Craig TJ, Goodman AB: Mortality in the era of deinstitutionalization. Am J Psychiatry 140:848–852, 1983

Hayward RSA, Steinberg EP, Ford DE, et al: Preventative care guidelines: 1991. Ann Intern Med 114:758–783, 1991

Hoyer EH, Mortensen PB, Olesen AV: Mortality and causes of death in a total national sample of patients with affective disorders admitted for the first time between 1973 and 1993. Br J Psychiatry 176:76–82, 2000

Jeste DV, Gladsjo JA, Lindamer LA, et al: Medical comorbidity in schizophrenia. Schizophr Bull 22:413–430, 1996

Jiang W, Alexander J, Christopher E, et al: Relationship of depression to increased risk of mortality and rehospitalization in patients with congestive heart failure. Arch Intern Med 161:1849–1856, 2001

Johnson NJ, Backlund E, Sorlie PD, et al: Marital status and mortality: the National Longitudinal Mortality Study. Ann Epidemiol 10:224–238, 2000

Josiassen RC, Schindler B: Medical comorbidity and schizophrenia: editors' introduction. Schizophr Bull 22:411–412, 1996

Kampmeier RH: Diagnosis and treatment of physical disease in mentally ill. Ann Intern Med 87:637–645, 1977

Katz IR, Streim J, Parmelee P: Psychiatric-medical comorbidity: implications for health services delivery and for research on depression. Biol Psychiatry 36:141–145, 1994

Kendell RE: The concept of disease and its implications for psychiatry. Br J Psychiatry 127:305–315, 1975

Kern DE, Roberts JC: Preventative medicine in ambulatory practice, in Ambulatory Medical Textbook, 4th Edition. Edited by Barker LR, Burton JR, Zieve P. Baltimore, MD, Williams & Wilkins, 1995, pp 17–29

Kligman EW, Hale FA: Clinical Prevention, in Family Medicine: Principles in Practice. Edited by Taylor RB. New York, Springer-Verlag, 1994, pp 29–52

Koran LM, Sox HC Jr, Marton KI, et al: Medical evaluation of psychiatric patients. Arch Gen Psychiatry 46:733–740, 1989

Koranyi EK: Physical health and illness in a psychiatric outpatient department population. Can Psychiatr Assoc J 17:109–116, 1972

Koranyi EK: Fatalities in 2070 psychiatric outpatients. Arch Gen Psychiatry 34:1137–1142, 1977

Koranyi EK: Morbidity and rate of undiagnosed physical illnesses in a psychiatric clinic population. Arch Gen Psychiatry 36:414–419, 1979

Lacro JP, Jeste DV: Physical comorbidity and polypharmacy in older psychiatric patients. Biol Psychiatry 36:146–152, 1994

Larson EB, Mack LA, Watts B, et al: Computed tomography in patients with psychiatric illnesses: advantages of a "rule in" approach. Ann Intern Med 95:360–364, 1981

Lawrence D, Holman CD, Jablensky AV, et al: Excess cancer mortality in Western Australian psychiatric patients due to higher case fatality rates. Acta Psychiatr Scand 101:382–388, 2000a

Lawrence D, Jablensky AV, Holman CD, et al: Mortality in Western Australian psychiatric patients. Soc Psychiatry Psychiatr Epidemiol 35:341–347, 2000b

Leeman CP: Diagnostic errors in emergency room medicine: physical illness in patients labeled "psychiatric" and vice versa. Int J Psychiatry Med 6:533–540, 1975

Lima BR, Pai S: Concurrent medical and psychiatric disorders among schizophrenic and neurotic outpatients. Community Ment Health J 23:30–39, 1987

Maes M, Bosmans E, Suy E, et al: Depression-related disturbances in mitogen-induced lymphocyte responses, interleukin-1B, and soluable interleukin-2 receptor production. Acta Psychiatr Scand 84:379–386, 1991

Martin RL, Preskorn SH: Use of the laboratory in psychiatry, in The Medical Basis of Psychiatry. Edited by Winokur G, Clayton P. Philadelphia, PA, WB Saunders, 1986, pp 522–540

Martin RL, Cloninger CR, Guze SB, et al: Mortality in a follow-up of 500 psychiatric outpatients, I: total mortality. Arch Gen Psychiatry 42:47–54, 1985a

Martin RL, Cloninger CR, Guze SB, et al: Mortality in a follow-up of 500 psychiatric outpatients, II: cause specific mortality. Arch Gen Psychiatry 42:58–66, 1985b

McIntyre JS, Romano J: Is there a stethoscope in the house (and is it used)? Arch Gen Psychiatry 34:1147–1151, 1977

Modrzewska K, Book JA: Schizophrenia and malignant neoplasms in a north Swedish population. Lancet I:275–276, 1979

Moos RH, Mertens JR: Patterns of diagnoses, comorbidities, and treatment in late-middle-aged and older affective disorder patients: comparison of mental health and medical sectors. J Am Geriatr Soc 44:682–688, 1996

Mortensen PB, Juel K: Mortality and causes of death in first admitted schizophrenic patients. Br J Psychiatry 163:183–189, 1993

Muecke LN, Krueger DW: Physical findings in a psychiatric outpatient clinic. Am J Psychiatry 138:1241–1242, 1981

Mueser KT, Bellack AS, Blanchard JJ: Comorbidity of schizophrenia and substance abuse: implications for treatment. J Consult Clin Psychol 60:845–856, 1992

Mukherjee S, Shukla J, Rosen A: Neurological abnormalities in patients with bipolar disorder. Biol Psychiatry 19:337–345, 1984

Murphy JM, Monson RR, Olivier DC, et al: Affective disorders and mortality. Arch Gen Psychiatry 44:473–480, 1987

Nasrallah HH, Tippin J, McCally Whitters M: Neurological soft signs in manic patients. J Affect Disord 5:45–50, 1983

Oken D, Fink PJ: General psychiatry: a primary-care specialty. JAMA 235:1973–1974, 1976

Parikh RM, Robinson RG, Lipsey JR, et al: The impact of post-stroke depression on recovery in activities of daily living over a 2-year follow-up. Arch Neurol 47:786–789, 1990

Patterson CW: Psychiatrists and physical examinations: a survey. Am J Psychiatry 135:967–968, 1978

Penninx BW, Beekman AT, Honig A, et al: Depression and cardiac mortality: results from a community-based longitudinal study. Arch Gen Psychiatry 58:221–227, 2001

Prager S, Jeste DV: Sensory impairment in late-life schizophrenia. Schizophr Bull 19:755–772, 1993

Regier DA, Farmer ME, Rae DS, et al: Comorbidity of mental disorders with alcohol and other drug abuse: results from the Epidemiological Catchment Area (ECA) study. JAMA 264:2511–2518, 1990

Roca RP, Breakey WR, Fischer PJ: Medical care of chronic psychiatric patients. Hosp Community Psychiatry 38:741–745, 1987

Rorsman B: Mortality among psychiatric patients. Acta Psychiatr Scand 50:354–375, 1974

Salazar-Fraile J, Gomez-Beneyto M, Perez-Hoyos S, et al: Mortality among psychiatric patients referred to the mental health services in Valencia. Soc Psychiatry Psychiatr Epidemiol 33:224–229, 1998

Saravay SM, Steinberg MD, Weinschel B, et al: Psychological comorbidity and length of stay in the general hospital. Am J Psychiatry 148:324–329, 1991

Saugstad LF, Odegard O: Mortality in psychiatric hospitals in Norway. Acta Psychiatr Scand 59:431–447, 1979

Savoca E: Psychiatric co-morbidity and hospital utilization in the general medical sector. Psychol Med 29:457–464, 1999

Schiffer RB, Klein RF, Sider RC: The Medical Evaluation of Psychiatric Patients. New York, Plenum, 1988, pp 15–17, 26–32, 35–76

Schleifer SJ, Macari-Hinson MM, Coyle DA, et al: The nature and course of depression following myocardial infarction. Arch Intern Med 149:1785–1789, 1989

Schwab B, Drake RE, Burghardt EM: Health care of the chronically mentally ill: the culture broker model. Community Ment Health J 24:174–184, 1988

Shekelle RB, Raynor WJ, Ostfeld Am, et al: Psychological depression and 17-year risk of death due to cancer. Psychosom Med 43:117–125, 1981

Sheline YI: High prevalence of physical illness in a geriatric psychiatric inpatient population. Gen Hosp Psychiatry 12:396–400, 1990

Simpson JC, Tsuang MT: Mortality among patients with schizophrenia. Schizophr Bull 22:485–499, 1996

Sims A: Mortality in psychiatric patients, in Physical Illness in the Psychiatric Patient. Edited by Koranyi EK. Springfield, IL, Charles C. Thomas, 1982, pp 24–41

Sims A: Why the excess mortality from psychiatric illness? Br Med J 294:986–987, 1987

Sohlman B, Lehtinen V: Mortality among discharged psychiatric patients in Finland. Acta Psychiatr Scand 99:102–109, 1999

Sox HC: Preventative health services in adults. N Engl J Med 330:1589–1595, 1994

Starkstein SE, Robinson RG: Affective disorders and cerebral vascular disease. Br J Psychiatry 154:170–182, 1989

Stein MB: Panic disorder and medical illness. Psychosomatics 27:833–838, 1986

Sternberg DE: Testing for physical illness in psychiatric patients. J Clin Psychiatry 47:3–9, 1986

Summers WK, Munoz RA: The psychiatric physical examination, part I: methodology. J Clin Psychiatry 42:95–98, 1981

Summers WK, Munoz RA, Read MR, et al: The psychiatric physical examination, part II: findings in 75 unselected psychiatric patients. J Clin Psychiatry 42:99–102, 1981

Talbott JA, Linn L: Reactions of schizophrenics to life threatening disease. Psychiatr Q 50:218–227, 1978

Thomas CJ: The use of screening investigations in psychiatry. Br J Psychiatry 135:67–72, 1979

Thorndike AN, Stafford RS, Rigotti NA: U.S. physicians' treatment of smoking in outpatients with psychiatric diagnoses. Nicotine Tob Res 3:85–91, 2001

Tishler PV, Woodward B, O'Connor, et al: High prevalence of intermittent acute porphyria in a psychiatric patient population. Am J Psychiatry 142:1430–1436, 1985

Torrey EF: Neurological abnormalities in schizophrenic patients. Biol Psychiatry 15:381–388, 1980

Tsuang MT, Woolson RF: Mortality in patients with schizophrenia, mania, depression and surgical conditions: a comparison with general population mortality. Br J Psychiatry 130:162–166, 1977

Tsuang MT, Woolson RF, Fleming JA: Causes of death in schizophrenia and manic depression. Br J Psychiatry 136:239–242, 1980

Tsuang MT, Perkins K, Simpson JC: Physical diseases in schizophrenia and affective disorder. J Clin Psychiatry 44:42–46, 1983

U.S. Preventative Services Task Force: Guide to clinical preventative services: Report of the U.S. Preventative Services Task Force. Baltimore, MD, Williams & Wilkins, 1989

von Ammon Cavanaugh S, Furlanetto LM, Creech SD, et al: Medical illness, past depression and present depression: a predictive triad for in-hospital mortality. Am J Psychiatry 158:43–48, 2001

Warnes H: Physical illness in the psychiatric patient, in Physical Illness in the Psychiatric Patient. Edited by Koranyi EK. Springfield, IL, Charles C. Thomas, 1982, pp 119–137

Weaver TE, Narsavage GL: Physiological and psychological variables related to functional status in chronic obstructive pulmonary disease. Nurs Res 41:286–291, 1992

Wells KB, Golding JM, Burnam MA: Chronic medical conditions in a sample of the general population with anxiety, affective, and substance use disorders. Am J Psychiatry 146:1440–1446, 1989

Winokur G, Black DW: Psychiatric and medical diagnoses as risk factors for mortality in psychiatric patients: a case-control study. Am J Psychiatry 144:208–211, 1987

Woods BT, Kinney DK, Yurgelun-Todd D: Neurological abnormalities in schizophrenic patients and their families, I: comparison of schizophrenic, bipolar, and substance abuse patients and normal controls. Arch Gen Psychiatry 43:657–663, 1986

Zilber N, Schufman N, Lerner Y: Mortality among psychiatric patients: the groups at risk. Acta Psychiatr Scand 79:248–256, 1989

Zubenko GS, Marino LJ, Sweet RA, et al: Medical comorbidity in elderly psychiatric inpatients. Biol Psychiatry 41:724–736, 1997

2

Reproductive Health

REPRODUCTIVE HEALTH NEEDS OF THE PATIENT WITH CHRONIC PSYCHIATRIC ILLNESS

Despite traditional misperceptions of chronic psychiatric patients as asexual persons, it is clear that many of these individuals are sexually active. Furthermore, improved medications for control of psychotic symptoms and consequent improved social function have led to increasing fertility rates in patients with schizophrenia and other serious mental illnesses (Trixler and Tenyi 1997). In addition to the reproductive health care required by all individuals, many psychiatric patients have unique reproductive health needs (Miller and Finnerty 1996; Rudolph et al. 1990). To date, these needs have remained poorly addressed. As a result, chronic psychiatric patients are at increased risk of coercive or abusive sexual relationships, rape and other sexual assaults, unplanned pregnancy, pregnancy complications, and sexually transmitted diseases (STDs) including HIV/AIDS (Coverdale and Aruffo 1992; Miller and Finnerty 1996; Seeman et al. 1990).

Reproductive health needs of chronic psychiatric patients include reproductive health maintenance, sex education, preventative services including counseling on safer sex, routine gynecologic and obstetrical care, contraception and family planning, and management of STDs including HIV infection (Table 2–1). Mental health care providers can optimize the health of chronically ill psychiatric patients by coordinating care with other providers to ensure that patients receive these services. Psychiatrists may choose to perform these services themselves or may defer them to other specialty physicians or physician extenders. In the latter case, the psychiatrist can play an important role by reviewing the care

Table 2–1. Reproductive health needs of chronic psychiatric patients

Health maintenance
Women
Routine gynecologic care (pelvic, Pap smear)
Breast examination, mammograms per guideline recommendations
Men
Testicular, prostate examination
Hepatitis B vaccine*
Education
Basic reproductive physiology
Menstrual hygiene/menopause
Sexual orientation/function/choices
Family planning/Obstetrics
Family planning/contraception services
Routine obstetrical care
Prenatal care
Delivery
Psychotropic drug management during pregnancy
Assessment of parenting skills
Management of unwanted pregnancy (abortion, adoption, support services)
Genetic counseling about risks of mental illness in offspring, potential teratogenicity of psychotropic drugs
Parenting classes
Preventative services
Counseling about sexually transmitted disease risk reduction, safe sex
Disease management
HIV/AIDS—prevention, diagnosis, treatment
Other sexually transmitted diseases—prevention, diagnosis, treatment
Rape—prevention, counseling, treatment

Note. *Hepatitis B vaccine is indicated for both men and women.

provided to ensure its completeness and appropriateness, as well as determining if there is a need for additional referrals.

REPRODUCTIVE HEALTH MAINTENANCE

Psychiatric patients require the same health maintenance care that is recommended for the general population. Routine gynecologic care for female patients should include pelvic examinations, Pap smears, breast examinations and instruction on breast self-examinations, and mammograms per the published guidelines. Women should have annual breast examinations starting at age 40 and mammography beginning at age 40–50. Pelvic examinations are indicated on an annual basis. Cervical cytologic screening (Pap smears) are recommended every 1–3 years. Instruction on the importance of self-examination of breasts and on the risks of unsafe sex are essential elements of medical counseling. Finally, the use of hormone replacement therapy should be discussed with all postmenopausal women. Male patients should receive prostate and testicular examinations as well as instruction on testicular self-examinations. Vaccination against hepatitis B should be offered to all high-risk individuals to interrupt sexual transmission of the illness.

Unfortunately, patients with chronic psychiatric illness are often unable to access medical health care for reproductive health maintenance because of barriers resulting directly from their mental illness as well as lack of insurance or erroneous impressions that their health needs will be met by their mental health care providers. Furthermore, practitioners may not provide needed services because of their belief that the physical examination or diagnostic testing may adversely affect the psychiatric condition, because of concern that the patient can not cooperate with such examinations, or because of negative attitudes that lead them to discriminate against the mentally ill. As an example, pelvic examinations are sometimes purposely omitted from the physical assessment of mentally ill women (Coverdale and Aruffo 1989; Coverdale et al. 1992; Handel 1985), allowing important and potentially life-threatening medical problems to be overlooked.

REPRODUCTIVE HEALTH EDUCATION

Sex education programs that address the special needs of the psychiatrically ill are urgently needed (Coverdale and Aruffo 1992; Miller and Finnerty 1996; Rudolph et al. 1990). Topics that could be taught include basic reproductive physiology, intimacy, sexuality, sexual orientation and preferences, contraception, STDs, pregnancy, labor and delivery, menstrual hygiene and menopause, the impact of psychotropic drugs on reproductive health, health screening, and parenting skills (Apfel and Handel 1993; Coverdale et al. 1997b; Seeman et al. 1990). Outpatient programs designed for chronic psychiatric patients and emphasizing sexual awareness (Pepper 1988) and sexual education and rehabilitation have been described (Coverdale and Aruffo 1992; Lukoff et al. 1986).

FAMILY PLANNING AND PREGNANCY

Contraception

Provision of contraception for the severely psychiatrically ill patient is critical but past abuses raise serious ethical and moral dilemmas for the practitioner (McCullough et al. 1992). It is important to remember that most patients with psychiatric problems, including many of those who are hospitalized, are sexually active and are in need of contraceptive advice. Patient autonomy must be respected by involving the patient in the decision-making process to the extent allowed by the mental illness (Coverdale et al. 1993). Past history of involuntary sterilization procedures has emphasized the importance of following legal guidelines when prescribing contraception (Egan et al. 1993).

Provision of contraception to patients who do not wish to become pregnant is critical to the overall management of psychiatrically ill patients (Apfel and Handel 1993). Condoms serve the dual purpose of protecting against STDs and preventing unwanted pregnancy (Coverdale and Aruffo 1989). However, chronic mentally ill women are often unable to successfully negotiate with their partners to use a condom, and the lack of female-controlled barrier protection is a major problem in ensuring adequate protection (Coverdale et al. 1995). Intrauterine devices, injectable medroxyprogesterone acetate, and tubal ligation may be preferred for patients unable or unwilling to use oral contraceptives or barrier methods. Psychotic patients may be suspicious or delusional about intrauterine devices (Casiano and Hawkins 1987; Coverdale et al. 1992) and may have altered pain thresholds that obscure the early signs of pelvic inflammatory disease due to the device (Coverdale and Aruffo 1989). Counseling the patient regarding the advantages and disadvantages of these options is an important responsibility of both the psychiatrist and the obstetrics and gynecology specialist. For patients with impaired autonomy, use of the least restrictive and, when possible, most reversible method of contraception is recommended (Egan et al. 1993).

Lack of access to family-planning services and failure to use contraception place many women with chronic psychiatric illnesses at risk for unwanted pregnancy (Coverdale and Aruffo 1989; Miller and Finnerty 1996). Patients with chronic psychiatric illness report that medical practitioners frequently fail to provide desired information on birth control (Coverdale and Aruffo 1989, 1992). Compared with women without chronic psychiatric illness, psychiatric patients are more likely to have induced abortions (Coverdale and Aruffo 1989; Coverdale et al. 1992). Furthermore, if they do complete the pregnancy, these women are more likely to give up their children for others to raise (Coverdale et al. 1997a;

Miller and Finnerty 1996). Male psychiatric patients are less likely than other men to use contraception and are often not involved in raising the children that they father (Coverdale et al. 1994, 1997b). Adverse outcomes are also more likely for the children conceived, with increased risk for various mental illnesses due to lack of consistent parenting, possible separation from their biological parents, and adverse socioeconomic conditions during childhood (Coverdale and Aruffo 1992; Coverdale et al. 1992). Finally, it has recently been recognized that traditional antipsychotic medications have a variety of endocrine side effects that may interfere with normal reproductive functioning. Hyperprolactinemia, amenorrhea, and infertility have been reported in women treated with these drugs (Currier and Simpson 1998a). The newer atypical antipsychotics such as clozapine and olanzapine are not associated with hyperprolactinemia. Patients should be counseled appropriately about these risks, and consultation with infertility experts may be advisable.

Obstetrical Care

Denial of pregnancy, feticide, and failure to obtain adequate prenatal and obstetrical care have been described among chronically ill psychiatric patients (Apfel and Handel 1993; Miller 1990). Studies indicate a correlation between the severity of the psychiatric disease and obstetrical complications (Miller 1992; Miller et al. 1990). Failure to receive good reproductive health care may be due to poor social functioning, low socioeconomic status, lack of education regarding the need for prenatal care, or lack of access to health care facilities (Casiano and Hawkins 1987). Furthermore, concern has been raised about possible adverse effects of some medications.

For patients wishing to become pregnant, a pre-pregnancy visit with an obstetrician familiar with the special needs of the chronically mentally ill should be encouraged. The visit should include a discussion of the risks to the mother and to the baby and a review of management of psychotropic drug therapy during the pregnancy. Once a woman becomes pregnant, consistent attendance at prenatal visits should be encouraged (Casiano and Hawkins 1987; Miller 1992). Careful collaboration between the obstetrician and psychiatrist can optimize the outcome for the mother, the baby, and the family unit (Apfel and Handel 1993).

Use of Psychotropic Drugs During Pregnancy

No psychotropic drugs have been approved for use during pregnancy (Altshuler et al. 1996), and the health care provider must be aware of the relative benefits and risks of the available agents for both mother and fetus (Apfel and Handel 1993; Briggs et al. 1994). Adverse effects fall into three categories: teratogenicity, perinatal syndromes (neonatal toxicity), and postnatal behavioral sequelae (Altshuler et al. 1996; Miller 1991; Walker et al. 1999) (Table 2–2). The decision to use psychotropic drugs should be reached by carefully weighing the risk of prenatal exposure against the risks to the fetus and mother posed by a relapse of the mother's psychiatric illness if drugs are withheld (Miller 1991).

Lithium

Lithium is teratogenic, and first-trimester exposure has been associated with an increased risk of Ebstein's anomaly (right ventricular hypoplasia, tricuspid insufficiency, and patent ductus arteriosus). The incidence in lithium-exposed children has been reported to be 0.1% (1 per 1,000), approximately 10- to 20-fold higher than in the general population (Altshuler et al. 1996; Cohen 1989; Cohen et al. 1989; Miller 1991). Controversy exists regarding whether lithium exposure increases the risk of other congenital abnormalities (Miller 1991). It is clear that use of lithium later in pregnancy can result in neonatal toxicity, manifested as neonatal goiter, poor sucking, impaired respiration, cardiac arrhythmia, reversible diabetes insipidus, and hypotonia with "floppy baby syndrome" (Cohen 1989; Cohen et al. 1989; Miller 1991).

Anticonvulsant Drugs

Anticonvulsants have been shown to be teratogenic when used to treat seizure disorders. The risks of these drugs when used for treatment of psychoses have not been thoroughly studied, although one would assume the same risks to be present. Carbamazepine has been considered to be a safer alternative than lithium for treatment of bipolar disorder during pregnancy (Cohen et al. 1989; Miller 1991). Although risk of neural tube defects and minor craniofacial anomalies has been suggested, the available studies indicate that this risk is quite low (Cohen et al. 1989; Miller 1991). Valproic acid has also been used for treatment of psychiatric illness. Exposure of the fetus to valproic acid has been associated with an incidence of spina bifida approximately 15 times greater than that observed in the general population (Altshuler et al. 1996). Orofacial clefts and a variety of minor malformations also appear to be increased in babies born to mothers taking valproic acid. Evidence supports the occurrence of a specific valproate syndrome after in utero exposure (Miller 1991). In addition, exposed infants may be developmentally delayed. Toxicity in the neonate can be manifested as liver problems and hyper-

Table 2–2. Use of psychotropic drugs during pregnancy

Drug class	FDA rating[a] by drug (representative trade name)	Risks[b,c]
Antianxiety agents	B: Buspirone (Buspar) C: Hydroxyzine (Atarax, Vistaril) D: Alprazolam (Xanax), chlordiazepoxide (Librium), clorazepate (Tranxene), diazepam (Valium), lorazepam (Ativan), meprobamate (Miltown), oxazepam (Serax)	The *Physician's Desk Reference* states that an increased risk of congenital malformations has been associated with the use of minor tranquilizers (chlordiazepoxide, diazepam, meprobamate) in first trimester, but further study is needed to define extent of risk. Specific anomaly most frequently associated with diazepam exposure was oral clefts, but recent studies fail to demonstrate increased risk. (?—behavioral teratogenicity). Exposed neonates have definite physiologic effects including hypotonia, lethargy, hypothermia, and apnea. Neonatal withdrawal syndrome is well documented.
Anti-insomnia agents	X: Flurazepam (Dalmane), temazepam (Restoril), triazolam (Halcion)	Use of these agents is contraindicated in pregnant women.
Antidepressants		
Monoamine oxidase inhibitors	C: Phenelzine (Nardil), tranylcypromine (Parnate)	Many experts recommend avoiding use of these drugs in pregnancy due to lack of studies.
Tricyclic antidepressants	C: Amoxapine (Asendin), desipramine (Norpramin), doxepin (Sinequan), protriptyline (Vivactil) D: Amitriptyline (Elavil), imipramine (Tofranil), nortriptyline (Pamelor)	Low risk of major teratogenic effects; however, more studies are needed to further explore early suggestions of various congenital malformations. Neonatal withdrawal symptoms include tachypnea, cyanosis, hypertonia, irritability, and seizure. Anticholinergic effects may cause urinary retention, bowel obstruction, or cardiac arrythmia. (Secondary amines such as nortriptyline and desipramine have fewer anticholinergic effects.)
Serotonin reuptake inhibitors	B: Fluoxetine (Prozac), paroxetine (Paxil) sertraline (Zoloft) C: Fluvoxamine (Luvox) D: Clomipramine (Anafranil)	Recent studies of fluoxetine suggest no increased risk of spontaneous pregnancy loss or major fetal anomalies. Use in third trimester may present increased risk for perinatal complications such as prematurity, respiratory difficulty, cyanosis, jitteriness, and low birth weight (Chambers et al. 1996).

Table 2–2. Use of psychotropic drugs during pregnancy *(continued)*

Drug class	FDA rating[a] by drug (representative trade name)	Risks[b,c]
Other	B: Bupropion (Wellbutrin), maprotiline (Ludiomil) C: Trazodone (Desyrel), nefazodone (Serzone), venlafaxine (Effexor)	
Antimania agents	D: Lithium	Lithium is not recommended in first trimester of pregnancy. Use of lithium during first trimester has been associated with risk of Ebstein's anomaly (tricuspid insufficiency, patent ductus arteriosus, right ventricle hypoplasia) at 0.1% (10–20 times general population) and other cardiac abnormalities. Risk of other congenital malformations is possible but less well established. Lithium toxicity can occur in neonate, leading to cyanosis, flaccidity, lethargy, reversible inhibition of thyroid function, cardiac arrythmias, and nephrogenic diabetes insipidus. (?—associated with prematurity). Use of lithium at time of delivery has been associated with impaired respiration, cardiac arrythmias, hypotonia in neonates. Use of lithium during nursing may result in hypertonia, hypothermia, cyanosis, and EKG changes in the baby.
	D: Valproic acid (Depakote)	Use of valproic acid has been associated with risk of teratogenicity, especially neural tube defects (?—specific fetal valproate syndrome). Do not combine with carbamazepine.
	C: Carbamazepine (Tegretol)	Carbamazepine may be a safer alternative to lithium for prophylaxis of bipolar disorder during early pregnancy. However, neural tube defects, minor craniofacial defects, and developmental delay may occur in exposed fetuses.

Table 2–2. Use of psychotropic drugs during pregnancy *(continued)*

Drug class	FDA rating[a] by drug (representative trade name)	Risks[b,c]
Antipsychotic agents	B: Clozapine (Clozaril) C: Chlorpromazine (Thorazine), fluphenazine (Prolixin), haloperidol (Haldol), loxapine (Loxitane), mesoridazine (Serentil), molindone (Moban), perphenazine (Trilafon), prochlorperazine (Compazine), risperidone (Risperdal), thioridazine (Mellaril), thiothixine (Navane), trifluoperazine (Stelazine)	Conflicting reports regarding teratogenicity—no definite link established but further studies are needed. Risk with low-potency drugs may be greater than for high-potency drugs. Use of antipsychotics has been associated with neonatal jaundice and extrapyramidal symptoms in infants after in utero exposure. Linkage has been suggested between respiratory depression, functional intestinal obstruction, and behavioral abnormalities and in utero exposure to antipsychotics.
Psychostimulants	C: Methylphenidate (Ritalin)	Possible increased risk of organ dysgenesis, especially oral clefts, but inconsistent study results. Neonatal withdrawal syndrome reported when mothers abuse amphetamines, but less well established when used for medical purposes.

Note. For all psychotropic drugs, the risk to the pregnant woman of withholding drugs must be balanced against the risk to the fetus/infant. All psychotropic drugs should be avoided in the first trimester if permitted by the mother's psychiatric condition.

[a]A = Controlled human studies fail to demonstrate risk to fetus in first trimester and possibility of fetal harm appears remote; B = Either animal studies have not demonstrated fetal risk but no human studies available, or animal studies show adverse effect but not confirmed in controlled human studies; C = Either animal studies demonstrate adverse effects on fetus and no human studies, or studies in animals and humans not available, therefore, drug should be given only if potential benefit justifies potential risk to fetus; D = Evidence of human fetal risk, but benefits from use in pregnant women may be acceptable despite risks (i.e., serious illness for which safer drugs are not available); X = Definite fetal risk and the risk of the use of the drug in pregnant women clearly outweighs any possible benefit.

[b]All psychotropic drugs, including benzodiazepines, antidepressants, lithium, and antipsychotics, are secreted in breast milk.

[c]Electroconvulsive therapy can be performed safely in pregnant women (Cohen 1989).

EKG = electrocardiogram; FDA = Food and Drug Administration.

glycemia (Miller 1991). The combination of valproic acid and carbamazepine is extremely teratogenic, and these drugs should not be used together during pregnancy.

Phenothiazines and Atypical Antipsychotics

Phenothiazines appear to be relatively safe for use during pregnancy (Cohen 1989). No definite link with congenital abnormalities has been established (Miller 1991). Nevertheless, most authorities recommend that phenothiazines be avoided in the first trimester whenever possible. High-potency antipsychotics may be safer than low-potency agents, based on the observation of possible teratogenicity in babies of mothers treated with low-potency agents for hyperemesis gravidarum (Altshuler et al. 1996; Cohen 1989; Cohen et al. 1989).

Phenothiazines should be discontinued several days before the estimated delivery date to decrease the risk of neonatal toxicity. Neonatal symptoms in exposed babies include jaundice, functional bowel obstruction, tremor, restlessness, respiratory depression, and difficulty with feeding. Significant extrapyramidal symptoms have been observed in neonates exposed in utero to phenothiazines (Miller 1991). Animal data have raised concern about the possibility of long-term behavioral sequelae in children exposed to antipsychotic drugs in utero, but to date, the limited studies have failed to definitively address these concerns (Cohen and Rosenbaum 1998; Trixler and Tenyi 1997; Walker et al. 1999).

Studies on the use of atypical antipsychotics during pregnancy are limited. It is now recognized that clozapine differs from traditional antipsychotics in that it does not cause hyperprolactinemia (Walker et al. 1999). As a result, fertility problems may be avoided. Successful pregnancy has been reported, although the possibility of a neonatal withdrawal syndrome has been posited (Currier and Simpson 1998b).

Tricyclic Antidepressants

Tricyclic antidepressants do not seem to significantly increase risk for organ dysgenesis (Altshuler et al. 1996; Miller 1991; Walker et al. 1999), and the use of these drugs appears to be relatively safe during pregnancy. Nevertheless, tricyclic antidepressant withdrawal syndromes have been observed in infants exposed to these medications during labor and delivery, manifested as tachypnea, cyanosis, hypertonia, jitteriness, irritability, convulsions, and anticholinergic symptoms including cardiac arrhythmias, functional bowel obstruction, and urinary retention (Miller 1991). If possible, discontinuing tricyclics about a week prior to delivery decreases the risk of withdrawal syndrome in the infant (Walker et al. 1999).

Doses of tricyclics may have to be adjusted during pregnancy to maintain therapeutic levels (Hostetter et al. 2000).

Selective Serotonin Reuptake Inhibitors/ Monoamine Oxidase Inhibitors

Data on the safety of selective serotonin reuptake inhibitors (SSRIs) during pregnancy are now starting to accumulate. Prenatal exposure to fluoxetine and other SSRIs appears to be safe (Kulin et al. 1998; Masand and Gupta 1999; Walker et al. 1999; Wisner et al. 1999). No increased risk of spontaneous pregnancy loss or major fetal anomalies was observed when women used the drug during pregnancy. However, one study found that women who took fluoxetine in the third trimester might be at increased risk of perinatal complications and that their babies might have problems such as feeding difficulties and jitteriness (Chambers et al. 1996). Other studies suggest that the drug is safe (Kulin et al. 1998; Walker et al. 1999; Wisner et al. 1999). Recent studies suggest that SSRI dosages may need to be increased during pregnancy to maintain euthymia (Hostetter et al. 2000). A recent study demonstrated that maternal levels of fluoxetine predict levels in nursing infants and that infant levels were low if women took less than 20 mg/day of fluoxetine (Hendrick et al. 2001). The risks of prenatal exposure to monoamine oxidase inhibitors are poorly defined (Miller 1991).

Psychostimulants

Psychostimulants such as methylphenidate are also occasionally used to treat depression. The use of prescribed psychostimulants has not been definitively shown to adversely affect outcomes of pregnancy (Altshuler et al. 1996); however, abuse of illicit amphetamines has been associated with growth retardation, premature delivery, increased congenital anomalies (especially oral clefts), perinatal syndromes of neonatal irritability, jerkiness, lassitude, and apnea, and possibly long-term behavioral alterations (Altshuler et al. 1996). Further studies will be necessary to determine if controlled medical use of psychostimulants is associated with similar complications.

Benzodiazepines

Exposure to benzodiazepines during the first trimester has been linked to a possible increased risk of congenital anomalies, especially oral clefts, but the extent of this risk remains controversial (Altshuler et al. 1996; Cohen 1989; Miller 1991). Adverse neonatal effects are reported in infants exposed to benzodiazepines in utero in the last trimester of pregnancy and at parturition, including hypotonicity, feeding problems, impaired temperature regulation, apnea, and low Apgar scores (Altshuler et al. 1996; Miller 1991). Neonatal withdrawal symptoms, including hypertonicity and irritability, and other behavioral changes have been reported. Animal studies suggest that exposure may be associated with long-term behavioral abnormalities, and further studies are warranted to determine if this risk occurs in humans as well.

Psychotropic Drug Management

Considering the risks of teratogenicity and neonatal toxicity posed by many psychoactive drugs, it is clear that careful attention must be paid to the appropriate use of psychotropics during pregnancy (Cohen et al. 1989; Miller 1991; Pinkofsky 2000; Wisner et al. 1999). However, the clinician must remember that there are risks to both mother and fetus in discontinuing antipsychotic medications. If the mother's psychosis worsens, she may develop delusions about the pregnancy and harm herself or the fetus (Cohen 1989). More commonly, a flare in psychotic symptoms may interfere with the mother's health (e.g., poor nutrition, poor hygiene) or prevent her from obtaining necessary medical treatment and prenatal care (Miller 1991). Therefore, the psychiatrist and obstetrician must work together with the patient to weigh the risks and benefits of using psychotropic drugs during pregnancy. The patient can then make an informed decision about the best course of action. Regardless of the choice, close monitoring of the mother's psychiatric condition, drug levels when appropriate, and possible side effects will be necessary throughout the pregnancy.

Management of the pregnant patient with bipolar disorder presents a major challenge (Miller 1991; Wisner et al. 1999). Discontinuation of lithium is clearly associated with a high rate of relapse, and the postpartum period may be a particularly high-risk time (Cohen et al. 1995). However, the risks of lithium use, especially during the first trimester, are well established. If possible, lithium should be discontinued prior to attempts at conception. Relapse of the bipolar disorder can constitute a medical emergency requiring aggressive intervention. Whenever possible, patients should be managed using antipsychotic medications, antidepressants, or electroconvulsive therapy (Cohen et al. 1989; Miller 1991; Wisner et al. 1999). If the mother's condition precludes discontinuing lithium, she should be counseled regarding the risks of lithium exposure to the developing fetus during the first trimester. Ultrasound of the fetus should be performed at week 16–20 (Cohen 1989; Cohen et al. 1989). If lithium is continued, it should be given in divided doses to minimize peak levels, and the dose should be tapered by 25%–50% just before delivery (Altshuler et al. 1996; Cohen 1989; Cohen et al. 1989; Miller 1991). If lithium is prescribed in the postpartum period, breast-feeding should be avoided because the drug is secreted into breast milk.

In some cases, consideration may be given to switching from lithium to an anticonvulsant such as carbamazepine or valproic acid (Cohen 1989; Cohen et al. 1989; Wisner et al. 1999), but this is controversial given the risks of these drugs (Miller 1991). If valproic acid is used, the woman must be counseled regarding the risks of neural tube defects. Ultrasound should be performed at week 16–19, amniocentesis with measurement of alpha-fetoprotein should be offered, and the importance of folate prophylaxis should be emphasized (Altshuler et al. 1996; Miller 1991).

Because the risks of agents used to control schizophrenia appear to be relatively low, most practitioners will continue the use of antipsychotics during pregnancy in patients with schizophrenia (Pinkofsky 2000). However, the dose should be minimized as much as possible, especially during the first trimester (Cohen 1989). Given observations of neonatal toxicity with lower-potency phenothiazines, higher-potency neuroleptics may be preferred. Some authorities state that it is generally not prudent to discontinue antipsychotic medications at the time of delivery (Altshuler et al. 1996), whereas others suggest tapering the drug prior to delivery if the mother's condition permits, with rapid reintroduction after delivery (Cohen 1989; Miller 1991).

Management of the patient with unipolar depression must be tailored to the severity of the patient's underlying disease. After counseling, some patients may elect to discontinue antidepressants, especially during the first trimester, if their symptoms are not severe (Cohen et al. 1989; Wisner et al. 1999). Alternative psychotherapeutic treatments such as cognitive therapy, interpersonal therapy, or, in some cases, light therapy may be adequate (Altshuler et al. 1996; Miller 1991). For patients requiring ongoing pharmacotherapy, SSRIs appear to be safe (Addis and Koren 2000; Kulin et al. 1998; Masand and Gupta 1999; Wisner et al. 1999) and are considered to be the best option for pregnant women in whom they are effective. Alternatively, secondary amine tricyclics with good safety profiles may be tried (Altshuler et al. 1996; Cohen et al. 1989). Secondary amines such as nortriptyline and desipramine may be preferable to more anticholinergic tertiary amines such as imipramine or amitriptyline (Cohen 1989; Miller 1991). If possible, tricyclic antidepressants should be tapered and discontinued prior to delivery to minimize neonatal withdrawal symptoms (Miller 1991). Careful monitoring of the mother for symptoms of recurrence or worsening of depression must accompany any medication change.

Electroconvulsive therapy (ECT) administered to pregnant women is usually not associated with dangers to the fetus (Cohen 1989). However, for depression near the time of delivery, it may be advisable to delay ECT until 4 weeks following childbirth. Several deaths have been reported with use of ECT in the puerperium, due to dislodging of deep venous thrombosis and consequent pulmonary embolism (Casiano and Hawkins 1987).

Because of the possible teratogenic risks associated with benzodiazepines, many practitioners will elect to attempt discontinuation of these drugs, especially during the first trimester of pregnancy (Cohen 1989; Cohen et al. 1989; Miller 1991). Alternative therapeutic strategies may be employed; the use of SSRIs or tricyclics for panic disorders (Altshuler et al. 1996; Miller 1991) or behavioral intervention for other anxiety disorders may be successful. Tapering of benzodiazepines prior to delivery will decrease the chances of neonatal withdrawal symptoms.

The psychotropics, including antipsychotics, antidepressants, and benzodiazepines, are secreted in breast milk. Although infants often are breast fed without adverse consequences by mothers taking psychotropic medications, many clinicians discourage nursing due to the possibility of neonatal toxicity and long-term sequalae in the exposed infants (Cohen 1989). In women with depression, lithium, fluoxetine, and doxepin should be used with caution. Fluoxetine has been associated with colic and doxepin with sedation in breast-fed infants (Ito 2000). Long-term use of diazepam and alprazolam should be avoided by women planning to breast-feed their babies (Ito 2000). Amitriptyline, nortriptyline, desipramine, and sertraline have not been detected in nurslings, suggesting that these agents may be considered the drugs of choice for women who elect to breast-feed their infants (Wisner et al. 1996).

Management of Unwanted Pregnancy

Unwanted pregnancy is a critical medical problem for the psychiatrically ill woman (Miller and Finnerty 1996). The risk of a flare in the psychiatric condition, including the development of delusions about the pregnancy, is real. The stress of pregnancy may prompt the woman to try harming the fetus or precipitate suicidal behavior. It is important that the mental health care provider identify the unwanted nature of the pregnancy and ensure referral to appropriate support services. The psychiatric condition should not prevent the mother from having access to the same variety of services available to all patients, including pregnancy support services, adoption, and abortion.

Parenting Skills

Mentally ill mothers are particularly vulnerable to parenting dysfunction and loss of custody of their children (Apfel and Handel 1993; Miller and Finnerty 1996; Nicholson et al. 1993). Even for those who retain custody, the stresses may exceed their coping skills, and their children are at high risk of poor social outcomes (Nicholson and Blanch 1974). Educational efforts to teach parenting skills to mentally ill mothers and fathers will benefit both parent and child (Coverdale et al. 1992; Miller and Finnerty 1996; Nicholson and Blanch 1974; Rudolph et al. 1990; Waldo et al. 1987).

RISK OF SEXUALLY TRANSMITTED DISEASES

Some patients with chronic psychiatric illnesses are particularly vulnerable to contracting STDs (Coverdale et al. 1995, 1997a, 1997b). As many as a third or more of patients with major psychoses report a history of treatment for STDs other than HIV (Kelly et al. 1992, 1995; Kim et al. 1992; Knox et al. 1994). Syphilis, gonorrhea, genital herpes, hepatitis B, hepatitis C, and *Chlamydia* infections (Rosenberg et al. 2001a, 2001b) are the major STDs that may occur in this patient population (Table 2–3).

Table 2–3. Major sexually transmitted diseases thought to occur with increased incidence in chronic psychiatric patients

HIV/AIDS	*Chlamydia* infections
Hepatitis B	Genital herpes
Syphilis	?—Papillomavirus
Gonorrhea	?—Other

Historical perceptions of the psychiatric patient as an asexual being clearly are not accurate. Indeed, some serious psychiatric conditions may be characterized by hypersexuality, especially organic brain syndrome and the manic phase of bipolar disorder (Cournos et al. 1994b; Tynes et al. 1993). Patients with personality disorders are likely to have had multiple sexual partners (Cournos et al. 1994b). Individuals with schizophrenia appear to have an initial increase in sexual activity that lessens over the course of the illness, with hyposexuality often characterizing late-stage disease (Brady and Carmen 1990; Cournos et al. 1994b). Importantly, when patients with schizophrenia are sexually active, they may engage in behaviors that place them at risk for HIV and other STDs (Cournos et al. 1994b). It is clear that fertility rates among women with schizophrenia are normal (Seeman et al. 1990). It must be acknowledged that many hospitalized psychiatric patients are sexually active and that even long-stay patients are at risk for acquiring HIV infection (American Psychiatric Association Commission on AIDS 1992, 1993; Meyer et al. 1993; Stefan and Catalan 1995).

Multiple factors put the patient with chronic psychiatric illness at risk for STDs (Table 2–4) (Coverdale et al. 1995).

Some chronically mentally ill patients may be at risk for STDs as a result of unsafe sexual behaviors (Rosenberg et al. 2001a). Cognitive impairment, due either to the mental illness itself or the drugs used to treat the condition, may hamper the patient's understanding of basic information regarding risks of STDs and preventative behaviors (Kelly et al. 1992; Tynes et al. 1993). Difficulty in evaluating the consequences of their decisions and impaired ability for long-range planning also place many chronic psychiatric patients at risk for acquisition of STDs.

Table 2–4. Postulated reasons for increased risk of HIV infection in chronic psychiatric patients

Unsafe sexual practices
Impaired cognitive understanding of risks of sexually transmitted diseases
Impaired appreciation of consequences of behavior
Poor impulse control
Self-destructive behavior/suicidal intent
Hypersexuality as manifestation of psychiatric illness (especially mania)
Poor interpersonal skills for negotiating safer sex practices
Substance abuse comorbidity
Sharing of potentially contaminated needles
Unsafe sexual behavior while intoxicated
Trading sex for drugs
Vulnerability of psychiatric patients to abuse, sexual exploitation
Other socioeconomic considerations—poverty, poor education, lack of support services, homelessness
Lack of access to education/counseling regarding risks of sexually transmitted diseases
Lack of access to health care for prevention/treatment of sexually transmitted diseases

HIV/AIDS IN THE PATIENT WITH CHRONIC PSYCHIATRIC ILLNESS

Risk of HIV

Patients with chronic psychiatric conditions are now known to represent a high-risk group for HIV infection and AIDS (Ayuso-Mateos et al. 1997;

Brady and Carmen 1990; Carey and Cournos 1997; Carmen and Brady 1990; Checkley et al. 1996; Chung et al. 1999; Cournos and Bakalar 1996; Cournos et al. 1994a; Davidson et al. 2001; Hellerstein and Prager 1992; Katz et al. 1994; Kelly et al. 1992, 1995; McDermott et al. 1994; McKinnon and Cournos 1997; McKinnon and Rosner 2000; Meyer et al. 1995; Naber et al. 1994; Perry et al. 1990; Sacks et al. 1990a, 1992; Schindler and Ferguson 1995; Seeman et al. 1990; Sullivan et al. 1999; Volavka et al. 1991). Studies of patients with bipolar disorder, schizophrenia, or severe depression have indicated HIV seroprevalence rates of 5%–20%, with the highest rates found among individuals with comorbid substance abuse, those who are homeless, and those living in certain urban areas in the United States (Cournos and McKinnon 1997; Empfield et al. 1993; Grassi 1996; Silberstein et al. 1994; Stefan and Catalan 1995; Stewart et al. 1994). Patients with personality disorders are also overrepresented among HIV-seropositive individuals (Brooner et al. 1993; Perkins et al. 1993). Other psychiatric disorders that have been associated with an increased risk of HIV include adolescent adjustment disorders (Baker and Mossman 1991; DiClemente and Ponton 1993; Stiffman et al. 1992) and alcoholism (Avins et al. 1994; Mahler et al. 1994).

Unfortunately, many mental health providers still fail to recognize that their patients are at high risk of exposure to HIV and therefore overlook the importance of incorporating HIV-related diagnostic and preventative measures into the health plan for their patients (Coverdale and Aruffo 1992; Grassi 1996; Hellerstein and Prager 1992; Ostrow 1992; Sullivan et al. 1999). Uneasiness in taking sexual histories, time pressures, concerns about the risk of worsening the psychopathology, fears about discrimination, and pessimism about efficacy of treatment measures have been cited as contributing to the failure to address HIV-related issues (Hellerstein and Prager 1992; Mahler et al. 1994). However, studies indicate that psychiatric patients often consider discussion of these issues to be less anxiety provoking and more desirable than do mental health providers (Coverdale and Aruffo 1992; Goisman et al. 1991; McKinnon et al. 1993). HIV risk assessment and counseling is a critical component of any psychiatric evaluation and care plan (Ostrow 1992; Sullivan et al. 1999).

Patients with chronic psychiatric conditions have a variety of risk factors for HIV infection (Carmen and Brady 1990; Cournos and McKinnon 1997; Coverdale and Turbott 2000; Kalichman et al. 1994; McKinnon 1996b; Sacks et al. 1992; Schindler and Ferguson 1995; Seeman et al. 1990; Tynes et al. 1993). Risky behaviors are practiced by a high proportion of psychiatric patients relative to the general population (McDermott et al. 1994; Menon et al. 1994). Classic risk factors for HIV include intravenous drug use, male-to-male sex, multiple sexual partners, blood transfusions received prior to 1985, and congenital transmission. Unsafe heterosexual activity, often in the context of unstable or transient relationships, appears to be the major risk behavior for HIV transmission among the chronically mentally ill (Cournos et al. 1993; Kalichman et al. 1994). Impulsivity, high levels of sexual activity during acute exacerbations of psychiatric illness, poor skills at negotiating safe sex, homelessness, and drug abuse are all HIV risk factors common among those affected by chronic, severe mental illnesses (Brady and Carmen 1990; Carmen and Brady 1990; Checkley et al. 1996; Sacks et al. 1992; Stewart et al. 1994; Tynes et al. 1993). Studies have repeatedly demonstrated distressingly infrequent use of condoms by chronically mentally ill patients (Kelly et al. 1995; Knox et al. 1994).

Comorbid substance abuse is high among patients with many psychiatric conditions, especially schizophrenia, personality disorder, and severe depression. Intravenous drug abuse is associated with a dramatically increased risk of exposure to blood-borne pathogens, including HIV and hepatitis B and C, due to sharing of contaminated needles (Ayuso-Mateos et al. 1997; Schneier and Siris 1987; Tynes et al. 1993). Abuse of drugs also increases the likelihood of participating in unsafe sexual practices when judgment is impaired by intoxication and because of the practice of trading sex for drugs. The role of crack cocaine in promoting the spread of HIV has been emphasized (Kim et al. 1992; Menon et al. 1994; Susser et al. 1995).

Psychiatric patients who engage in unsafe sex practices do so for many reasons (Cates and Graham 1993; Cournos et al. 1991; Naber et al. 1994; Sacks et al. 1990a; Schindler and Ferguson 1995; Seeman et al. 1990). The mental illness may result in cognitive dysfunction that interferes with the ability to understand the factual information necessary to accurately assess HIV risk, to perceive when behavior entails risk for HIV, or to learn about protective practices (Brady and Carmen 1990; Carmen and Brady 1990; Katz et al. 1994). Patients with severe, chronic psychiatric illnesses may significantly underestimate the HIV risk of behaviors in which they engage (Knox et al. 1994), and their fund of knowledge regarding HIV is significantly smaller than that of the general population (Aruffo et al. 1990; Grassi et al. 2001; McDermott et al. 1994; Menon et al. 1994; Steiner et al. 1992; Tynes et al. 1993). Psychiatric illness may be directly linked to hypersexuality as sometimes observed in mania or may result in impaired decision-making practices due to lack of impulse control or depression (Sacks et al. 1990a, 1990b). Other psychiatric patients may be at risk because their illness makes them more vulnerable to abusive relationships or coercion into unwanted sexual liaisons (Grassi 1996; Kelly et al. 1995). Finally, chronically mentally ill patients, especially those with schizophrenia and other major psychoses, are more likely to be of lower socioeconomic status and thus have less access to health care counseling or treatment facilities (Steiner et al. 1992). The homeless represent a population at particular risk for psychiatric illness, substance abuse, and HIV infection (Brady and Carmen 1990; Checkley et al. 1996; Susser et al. 1993, 1995; Tynes et al. 1993).

Identification of HIV-Infected Patients

Studies of medical records reveal that information on risk behaviors is often not noted by the mental health provider (Cournos et al. 1991; Hellerstein and Prager 1992; Mahler et al. 1994; McKinnon 1996a; Menon et al. 1994; Sacks et al. 1992) and that many psychiatric patients are discharged from the hospital without identification of their HIV status (Silberstein et al. 1994). Unfortunately, reluctance by health providers to embark on sexual history taking and counseling of the mentally ill is well documented (Brady and Carmen 1990; Checkley et al. 1996; Menon et al. 1994). Questionnaires have been developed that facilitate identification of chronic mentally ill patients at risk for HIV infection and AIDS (Brady and Carmen 1990; Volavka et al. 1992). However, even when risk factors are identified, many mental health care practitioners fail to counsel the patient and order HIV testing (Brady and Carmen 1990; Sacks et al. 1992; Walkup et al. 1998), resulting in missed opportunities to initiate early treatment or educate patients to interrupt further transmission (Sullivan et al. 1999; Walkup et al. 2000).

Prevention and Education

Programs to address HIV risk in the chronically ill psychiatric patient require appropriate educational and preventative services as well as diagnostic and treatment services that address the special needs of these patient populations (Table 2–5).

Preventative programs that specifically target the unique needs of patients with chronic mental illnesses are desirable (Ayuso-Mateos et al. 1997; Brady and Carmen 1990; Cates and Graham 1993; Goisman et al. 1991; Kalichman et al. 1995; Katz et al. 1994; McDermott et al. 1994; Menon et al. 1994; Meyer et al. 1995; Schindler and Ferguson 1995; Sladyk 1990; Sullivan et al. 1999; Tynes et al. 1993). Education of patients with chronic psychoses must include remediation of their lack of knowledge regarding HIV (Aruffo et al. 1990; Carmen and Brady 1990; Goisman et al. 1991; Grassi 1996; Kalichman et al. 1995; Katz et al. 1994; Sacks et al. 1991; Steiner et al. 1992). Educational programs must consider the educational background and social experiences of the chronically ill psychi-

Table 2–5. Approaches to prevention, diagnosis, and management of HIV infection in chronic psychiatric patients

Recommended
Prevention and education
History to identify high-risk behaviors
HIV risk reduction/educational programs tailored to the needs of psychiatric patient populations (both inpatient and outpatient)
Improved access to substance abuse programs
Improved access to family planning/contraception services
Use of "standard" precautions in all health care settings
Diagnosis and management
History and physical examination to detect symptoms/signs of HIV infection
HIV antibody testing (ELISA/Western blot) in patients with identified risk factors
Referral of HIV-infected patients to physician with expertise in HIV as soon as diagnosis is made
Provision of HIV testing and pre- and post-test counseling in psychiatric facilities
Controversial
Needle exchange programs
Not recommended
Routine testing of all psychiatric patients
Special isolation procedures for patients with HIV infection

Note. ELISA= enzyme-linked immunosorbent assay.

atric patient and compensate for possible cognitive impairment (Grassi 1996). Counseling on risk reduction must occur at a pace that is consistent with the patient's ability to understand and must be tailored to the patient's psychiatric condition (Hajagos et al. 1998; Kalichman et al. 1995). Patients should be empowered to make judicious choices about their sexuality and their sexual behavior. Communication skills (e.g., how to say "no," how to negotiate in a sexual relationship) and the proper use of contraception can be taught. Practical skills such as the use of condoms (how to buy them and put them on) are also important components of education (Brady and Carmen 1990; Carmen and Brady 1990; Knox et al. 1994).

Components of HIV prevention programs for patients with severe, chronic psychiatric illnesses should include the following:

- Factual information on HIV risk factors and availability of testing
- Specific training on behavioral techniques to reduce HIV risk, including safer sex and use of condoms

- Role playing to provide the necessary interpersonal skills for empowering patients to successfully identify appropriate sexual relationships and negotiate safe sex practices

A variety of HIV education programs have been developed to serve chronically ill psychiatric patients (American Psychiatric Association Commission on AIDS 1992; Baer et al. 1988; Brady and Carmen 1990; Carmen and Brady 1990; Goisman et al. 1991; Graham and Cates 1992; Katz et al. 1996; Miller and Finnerty 1996; Otto-Salaj et al. 1996). It is clear that programs can be designed that do not aggravate the psychiatric condition (Goisman et al. 1991; Grassi 1996). Unfortunately, these educational and counseling services have not been adopted by most psychiatric facilities (McKinnon et al. 1999), presumably because many practitioners perceive them to be outside the purview of the mental health provider. Recent work has suggested that such services are best delivered when provided by or at least coordinated with the mental health facility (Ayuso-Mateos et al. 1997; Silberstein et al. 1994; Tate and Longo 2000). Offering comprehensive family planning and STD prevention services in the psychiatric hospital or clinic has been recommended as an effective first step in providing improved access to this information for patients with chronic psychiatric illnesses (Coverdale et al. 1995; Menon et al. 1994; Seeman et al. 1990).

Diagnosis and Management

Routine HIV testing of all psychiatric patients is not appropriate (American Psychiatric Association Commission on AIDS 1992, 1993; Cournos et al. 1989; Naber et al. 1994). However, all mental health providers should incorporate identification of risk factors into their clinical patient assessments (Ayuso-Mateos et al. 1997; Brady and Carmen 1990; Grassi 1996; Kelly et al. 1992; Stewart et al. 1994). A history that includes information on substance abuse and sexual behaviors should be an accepted part of the assessment and treatment of all patients, including those with psychiatric conditions (Checkley et al. 1996). Protocols have been developed to assist the mental health practitioner in this endeavor (Brady and Carmen 1990; Volavka et al. 1992). Furthermore, psychiatric facilities should be prepared to perform pre- and post-test counseling and confidential HIV testing when risk factors are identified (American Psychiatric Association Commission on AIDS 1992, 1993; Carlson et al. 1989; Checkley et al. 1996; Oquendo and Tricarico 1996; Stewart et al. 1994). Early identification of patients with HIV infection will allow appropriate referrals so that the patient can receive counseling, prophylaxis against opportunistic infections, and antiretroviral therapies that have now been demonstrated to prolong survival and improve quality of life (Kramer 1996). Practice guidelines for the treatment of patients with HIV/AIDS have recently been published by the American Psychiatric Association (Work Group on HIV/AIDS 2000).

Infection Control in Health Care Settings

In health care settings, infection-control policies that prevent contact with blood and other bodily substances capable of transmitting blood-borne pathogens, termed "universal" or "standard" precautions, should be followed when caring for all patients; special precautions with patients known to be HIV seropositive are not indicated. "Standard precautions" include careful hand washing, use of gloves when handling or coming into contact with blood and other body substances, and use of appropriate personal protective equipment (e.g., gowns, safety glasses, masks) when performing procedures that entail potential exposure to blood and body substances. Only by considering all patients as potentially infected can optimal protection of staff and other patients be achieved. If a health care worker is exposed to blood or other body substances that are capable of transmitting blood-borne pathogens, immediate evaluation by a practitioner familiar with occupational exposures should be undertaken. Published guidelines emphasize the role of prompt initiation of antiretroviral prophylaxis to health care workers with high-risk occupational exposure, as well as counseling and serologic monitoring (http://www.hivatis.org).

SEXUAL ASSAULT AND RAPE

Many chronically mentally ill patients are at increased risk of sexual exploitation and sexual assault, including rape (Coverdale et al. 1995; Miller and Finnerty 1996). Studies indicate that many severely ill psychiatric patients have been victims of a major physical and/or sexual assault and that mental health care providers frequently fail to ascertain this history (Jacobson and Richardson 1987; Miller and Finnerty 1996). Both male and female patients appear to be at risk for sexual assault, and men may be particularly reluctant to reveal the assault experience to their therapists. Clearly, assault places the patient at risk of STDs including HIV infection. Furthermore, these experiences impose additional psychiatric stresses that increase the chances for future sexual exploitation and interfere with optimal psychosocial adjustment. Prevention programs that teach behavioral skills for avoiding unwanted sexual advances and that offer rape prevention classes will be of benefit to chronic psychiatric patients. Treatment of assault and rape victims by health care providers familiar with the needs of chronically ill psychiatric patients is desirable.

SUMMARY

Patients with chronic psychiatric illness have a variety of reproductive health needs and are at increased risk for several reproductive health complications. Reproductive health maintenance, sex education programs, family planning and obstetrical services, and prevention and management of rape, assault, and STDs including HIV are of vital importance to the total health care of psychiatric patients. Unfortunately, these needs often remain unaddressed. Practitioners caring for these vulnerable populations should strive to ensure that their patients are able to access these services when appropriate.

REFERENCES

Addis A, Koren G: Safety of fluoxetine during the first trimester of pregnancy: a meta-analytical review of epidemiological studies. Psychol Med 30:89–94, 2000

Altshuler LL, Cohen L, Szuba MP, et al: Pharmacological management of psychiatric illness during pregnancy: dilemmas and guidelines. Am J Psychiatry 153:592–606, 1996

American Psychiatric Association Commission on AIDS: AIDS policy: guidelines for outpatient psychiatry services. Am J Psychiatry 149:721, 1992

American Psychiatric Association Commission on AIDS: AIDS policy: guidelines for inpatient psychiatric units. Am J Psychiatry 150:853, 1993

Apfel RJ, Handel MH: Madness and Loss of Motherhood: Sexuality, Reproduction, and Long-Term Mental Illness. Washington, DC, American Psychiatric Press, 1993

Aruffo JF, Coverdale JH, Chacko RC, et al: Knowledge about AIDS among women psychiatric outpatients. Hosp Community Psychiatry 41:326–328, 1990

Avins AL, Woods WJ, Lindan CO, et al: HIV infection and risk behaviors among heterosexuals in alcohol treatment programs. JAMA 271:515–518, 1994

Ayuso-Mateos JL, Montanes F, Lastra I, et al: HIV infection in psychiatric patients: an unlinked anonymous study. Br J Psychiatry 170:181–185, 1997

Baer JW, Dwyer PC, Lewitter-Koehler S: Knowledge about AIDS among psychiatric patients. Hosp Community Psychiatry 39:986–988, 1988

Baker DG, Mossman D: Potential HIV exposure in psychiatrically hospitalized adolescent girls. Am J Psychiatry 148:528–530, 1991

Brady SM, Carmen E: AIDS risk in the chronically mentally ill: clinical strategies for prevention. New Directions for Mental Health Services 48:83–95, 1990

Briggs G, Freeman R, Yaffe S: Drugs in Pregnancy and Lactation, 4th Edition, Baltimore, MD, Williams & Wilkins, 1994

Brooner RK, Greenfield L, Schmidt CW, et al: Antisocial personality disorder and HIV infection among intravenous drug abusers. Am J Psychiatry 150:53–58, 1993

Carey MP, Cournos F: HIV and AIDS among the severely mentally ill: introduction to the special series. Clin Psychol Rev 17:241–245, 1997

Carlson GA, Greenman M, McClellan TA: Management of HIV-positive psychiatric patients who fail to reduce high risk behaviors. Hosp Community Psychiatry 40:511–514, 1989

Carmen E, Brady SM: AIDS risk and prevention for the chronically mental ill. Hosp Community Psychiatry 41:652–657, 1990

Casiano ME, Hawkins DR: Major mental illness and childbearing. Psychiatr Clin North Am 10:35–51, 1987

Cates JA, Graham LL: HIV and serious mental illness: reducing the risk. Community Ment Health J 29:35–47, 1993

Chambers CD, Johnson KA, Dick LM, et al: Birth outcomes in pregnant women taking fluoxetine. N Engl J Med 335:1010–1015, 1996

Checkley GE, Thompson SC, Crofts N, et al: HIV in the mentally ill. Australia and New Zealand Journal of Psychiatry 30:184–194, 1996

Chung JY, Suarez AP, Zarin DA, et al: Datapoints: psychiatric patients and HIV. Psychiatr Serv 50:487–490, 1999

Cohen LS: Psychotropic drug use in pregnancy. Hosp Community Psychiatry 40:566–567, 1989

Cohen L, Rosenbaum J: Psychotropic drug use during pregnancy: weighing the risks. J Clin Psychiatry 59:18–28, 1998

Cohen LS, Heller VL, Rosenbaum JF: Treatment guidelines for psychotropic drug use in pregnancy. Psychosomatics 30:25–33, 1989

Cohen LS, Sichel DA, Robertson BA, et al: Postpartum prophylaxis for women with bipolar disorder. Am J Psychiatry 152:1641–1645, 1995

Cournos F, Bakalar N: AIDS and People With Severe Mental Illness. New Haven, CT, Yale University Press, 1996

Cournos F, McKinnon K: HIV seroprevalence among people with severe mental illness in the United States: a critical review. Clin Psychol Rev 17:259–269, 1997

Cournos F, Empfield M, Horwath E, et al: The management of HIV infection in state psychiatric hospitals. Hosp Community Psychiatry 40:153–157, 1989

Cournos F, Empfield M, Horwath E, et al: HIV seroprevalence among patients admitted to two psychiatric hospitals. Am J Psychiatry 148:1225–1230, 1991

Cournos F, Horwath E, Guido JR, et al: HIV-1 infection at two public psychiatric hospitals in New York City. AIDS Care 6:443–452, 1994a

Cournos F, Guido JR, Coomaraswamy S: Sexual activity and risk of HIV infection among patients with schizophrenia. Am J Psychiatry 151:228–232, 1994b

Cournos F, McKinnon K, Meyer-Bahlburg H, et al: HIV risk activity among persons with severe mental illness: preliminary findings. Hosp Community Psychiatry 44:1104–1106, 1993

Coverdale JH, Aruffo J: Family planning needs of female chronic psychiatric outpatients. Am J Psychiatry 146:1489–1491, 1989

Coverdale JH, Aruffo J: AIDS and family planning counseling of psychiatrically ill women in community mental health clinics. Community Ment Health J 28:13–20, 1992

Coverdale JH, Turbott SH: Risk behaviors for sexually transmitted infections among men with mental disorders. Psychiatr Serv 51:234–238, 2000

Coverdale JH, Aruffo J, Grunebaum H: Developing family planning services for female chronic mentally ill outpatients. Hosp Community Psychiatry 43:475–478, 1992

Coverdale JH, Bayer TL, McCullough LB, et al: Respecting the autonomy of chronic mentally ill women in decisions about contraception. Hosp Community Psychiatry 44:671–674, 1993

Coverdale JH, Schotte D, Ruiz P, et al: Family planning needs of male chronic mental patients in the general hospital psychiatry clinic. Gen Hosp Psychiatry 16:38–41, 1994

Coverdale JH, Bayer TL, McCullough LB, et al: Sexually transmitted disease prevention services for female chronically mentally ill patients. Community Ment Health J 31:303–315, 1995

Coverdale JH, Turbott SH, Roberts H: Family planning and STD risk behaviours of female psychiatric out-patients. Br J Psychiatry 171:69–72, 1997a

Coverdale JH, McCullough LB, Chervenak FA: Sexually transmitted diseases and unwanted pregnancies in chronically ill psychiatric patients. Med J Aust 166:231–232, 1997b

Currier GW, Simpson GM: Antipsychotic medications and fertility. Psychiatr Serv 49:175–176, 1998a

Currier GW, Simpson GM: Pregnancy and clozapine. Psychiatr Serv 49:997, 1998b

Davidson S, Judd F, Jolley D, et al: Risk factors for HIV/AIDS and hepatitis C among the chronic mentally ill. Aust N Z J Psychiatry 35:203–209, 2001

DiClemente RJ, Ponton LE: HIV-related risk behavior among psychiatrically hospitalized adolescents and school-based adolescents. Am J Psychiatry 150:324–325, 1993

Egan TM, Siegert RJ, Fairley NA: Use of hormonal contraceptives in an institutional setting: reasons for use, consent and safety in women with psychiatric and intellectual disabilities. N Z Med J 106:338–341, 1993

Empfield M, Cournos F, Meyer I, et al: HIV seroprevalence among homeless patients admitted to a psychiatric inpatient unit. Am J Psychiatry 150:47–52, 1993

Goisman RM, Kent AB, Montgomery EC: AIDS education for patients with chronic mental illness. Community Ment Health J 27:189–197, 1991

Graham LL, Cates JA: How to reduce the risk of HIV infection for the seriously mentally ill. J Psychosoc Nurs Ment Health Serv 30:9–13, 1992

Grassi L: Risk of HIV infection in psychiatrically ill patients. AIDS Care 8:103–116, 1996

Grassi L, Biancosino B, Righi R, et al: Knowledge about HIV transmission and prevention among Italian patients with psychiatric disorders. Psychiatr Serv 52:679–681, 2001

Hajagos K, Geiser P, Parker B, et al: Safer-sex education for persons with mental illness. J Psychosoc Nurs Ment Health Serv 36:33–37, 1998

Handel M: Deferred pelvic examinations: a purposeful omission in the care of mentally ill women. Hosp Community Psychiatry 36:1070–1074, 1985

Hellerstein DJ, Prager ME: Assessing HIV risk in the general hospital psychiatric clinic. Gen Hosp Psychiatry 14:3–6, 1992

Hendrick V, Stowe ZN, Altshuler LL, et al: Fluoxetine and norfluoxetine concentrations in nursing infants and breast milk. Biol Psychiatry 50:775–782, 2001

Hostetter A, Stowe ZN, Strader JR Jr, et al: Dose of selective serotonin reuptake inhibitors across pregnancy: clinical implications. Depress Anxiety 11:51–57, 2000

Ito S: Drug therapy for breast-feeding women. N Engl J Med 343:118–126, 2000

Jacobson A, Richardson B: Assault experiences of 100 psychiatric inpatients: evidence of the need for routine inquiry. Am J Psychiatry 144:908–912, 1987

Kalichman SC, Kelly JA, Johnson JR, et al: Factors associated with risk for HIV infection among chronic mentally ill adults. Am J Psychiatry 151:221–227, 1994

Kalichman SC, Sikkema KJ, Kelly JA, et al: Use of a brief behavioral skills intervention to prevent HIV infection among chronically mentally ill adults. Psychiatr Serv 46:275–280, 1995

Katz RC, Watts C, Santman J: AIDS knowledge and high risk behaviors in the chronic mentally ill. Community Ment Health J 30:395–402, 1994

Katz RC, Westerman C, Beauchamp K, et al: Effects of AIDS counseling and risk reduction training on the chronic mentally ill. AIDS Education and Prevention 8:457–463, 1996

Kelly JA, Murphy DA, Bahr R, et al: AIDS/HIV risk behavior among chronic mentally ill. Am J Psychiatry 149:886–889, 1992

Kelly JA, Murphy DA, Sikkema KJ, et al: Predictors of high and low levels of HIV risk behavior among adults with chronic mental illness. Psychiatr Serv 46:813–818, 1995

Kim A, Galanter M, Castaneda R, et al: Crack cocaine use and sexual behavior among psychiatric inpatients. Am J Drug Alcohol Abuse 18:235–246, 1992

Knox MD, Boaz TL, Friedrich MA, et al: HIV risk factors for persons with serious mental illness. Community Ment Health J 30:551–563, 1994

Kramer M: Medical manifestations, in AIDS and People With Severe Mental Illness. Edited by Cournos F, Bakalar N. New Haven, CT, Yale University Press, 1996, pp 74–94

Kulin NA, Pastuszak A, Sage SR, et al: Pregnancy outcome following maternal use of the new selective serotonin reuptake inhibitors: a prospective controlled multicenter study. JAMA 279:609–610, 1998

Lukoff D, Giola-Hasick D, Sullivan G: Sex education and rehabilitation with schizophrenic male outpatients. Schizophr Bull 12:669–677, 1986

Mahler J, Yi D, Sacks M, et al: Undetected HIV infection among patients admitted to an alcohol rehabilitation unit. Am J Psychiatry 151:439–440, 1994

Masand PS, Gupta S: Selective serotonin reuptake inhibitors: an update. Harv Rev Psychiatry 7:69–84, 1999

McCullough LB, Coverdale JH, Bayer T: Ethically justified guidelines for family planning interventions to prevent pregnancy in female patients with chronic mental illness. Am J Obstet Gynecol 167:19–25, 1992

McDermott BE, Sautter FJ, Winstead DK: Diagnosis, health beliefs, and risk of HIV infection in psychiatric patients. Hosp Community Psychiatry 45:580–585, 1994

McKinnon K: Risk behavior assessment, in AIDS and People With Severe Mental Illness. Edited by Cournos F, Bakalar N. New Haven, CT, Yale University Press, 1996a, pp 47–56

McKinnon K: Sexual and drug-use risk behavior, in AIDS and People With Severe Mental Illness. Edited by Cournos F, Bakalar N. New Haven, CT, Yale University Press, 1996b, pp 17–46

McKinnon K, Cournos F: Research on HIV, AIDS and severe mental illness: recommendations from the NIMH National Conference. Clin Psychol Rev 17:327–331, 1997

McKinnon K, Rosner J: Severe mental illness and HIV-AIDS. New Dir Ment Health Serv Fall:69–76, 2000

McKinnon K, Cournos F, Meyer-Bahlburg HFL, et al: Reliability of sexual risk behavior interviews with psychiatric patients. Am J Psychiatry 150:972–974, 1993

McKinnon K, Cournos F, Herman R, et al: AIDS-related services and training in outpatient mental health care agencies in New York. Psychiatr Serv 50:1225–1228, 1999

Menon AS, Pomerantz S, Harowitz S, et al: The high prevalence of unsafe sexual behaviors among acute psychiatric inpatients: implications for AIDS prevention. J Nerv Ment Dis 182:661–666, 1994

Meyer I, McKinnon K, Cournos F, et al: HIV seroprevalence among long-stay patients in a state psychiatric hospital. Hosp Community Psychiatry 44:282–284, 1993

Meyer I, Empfield M, Engel D, et al: Characteristics of HIV-positive chronically mentally ill patients. Psychiatr Q 66:201–207, 1995

Miller LJ: Psychotic denial of pregnancy: phenomenology and clinical management. Hosp Community Psychiatry 41:1233–1237, 1990

Miller LJ: Clinical strategies for the use of psychotropic drugs during pregnancy. Psychiatr Med 9:275–298, 1991

Miller LJ: Comprehensive care of pregnant mentally ill women. J Ment Health Adm 19:170–177, 1992

Miller LJ, Finnerty M: Sexuality, pregnancy, and childrearing among women with schizophrenia-spectrum disorders. Psychiatr Serv 47:502–506, 1996

Miller WH, Resnick MP, Williams MH: The pregnant psychiatric inpatient: a missed opportunity. Gen Hosp Psychiatry 12:373–378, 1990

Naber D, Pajonk FG, Perro C: Human immunodeficiency virus antibody test and seroprevalence in psychiatric patients. Acta Psychiatr Scand 89:358–361, 1994

Nicholson J, Blanch A: Rehabilitation for parenting roles for people with serious mental illness. Psychosocial Rehabilitation Journal 18:109–119, 1974

Nicholson J, Geller JL, Fisher WH, et al: State policies and programs that address the needs of mentally ill mothers in the public sector. Hosp Community Psychiatry 44:484–489, 1993

Oquendo M, Tricarico P: Pre- and post-HIV test counseling, in AIDS and People With Severe Mental Illness. Edited by Cournos F, Bakalar N. New Haven, CT, Yale University Press, 1996, pp 97–112

Ostrow DG: HIV counseling and testing of psychiatric patients: time to reexamine policy and practices. Gen Hosp Psychiatry 14:1–2, 1992

Otto-Salaj LL, Stevenson Y, Kelly JA: Risk reduction strategies, in AIDS and People With Severe Mental Illness. Edited by Cournos F, Bakalar N. New Haven, CT, Yale University Press, 1996, pp 113–124

Pepper E: Sexual awareness groups in a psychiatric day treatment program. Psychosocial Rehabilitation Journal 11:45–52, 1988

Perkins DO, Davidson EJ, Leserman J, et al: Personality disorder in patients infected with HIV: a controlled study with implications for clinical care. Am J Psychiatry 150:309–315, 1993

Perry S, Jacobsberg LB, Fishman B, et al: Psychiatric diagnosis before serological testing for the human immunodeficiency virus. Am J Psychiatry 147:89–93, 1990

Pinkofsky HB: Effects of antipsychotics on the unborn child: what is known and how should this influence prescribing? Paediatr Drugs 2:83–90, 2000

Rosenberg SD, Trumbetta SL, Mueser KT, et al: Determinants of risk behavior for human immunodeficiency virus/acquired immunodeficiency syndrome in people with severe mental illness. Compr Psychiatry 42:263–271, 2001a

Rosenberg SD, Goodman LA, Osher FC, et al: Prevalence of HIV, hepatitis B, and hepatitis C in people with severe mental illness. Am J Public Health 91:31–37, 2001b

Rudolph B, Larson GL, Sweeny S, et al: Hospitalized pregnant psychotic women: characteristics and treatment issues. Hosp Community Psychiatry 41:159–162, 1990

Sacks M, Silberstein C, Weiler P, et al: HIV-related risk factors in acute psychiatric inpatients. Hosp Community Psychiatry 41:449–451, 1990a

Sacks M, Perry S, Graver R, et al: Self-reported HIV-related risk behaviors in acute psychiatric inpatients: a pilot study. Hosp Community Psychiatry 41:1253–1255, 1990b

Sacks M, Dermatis H, Looser-Ott S, et al: Undetected HIV infection among acutely ill psychiatric inpatients. Am J Psychiatry 149:544–545, 1991

Sacks M, Dermatis H, Looser-Ott S, et al: Seroprevalence of HIV and risk factors for AIDS in psychiatric inpatients. Hosp Community Psychiatry 43:736–737, 1992

Schindler VP, Ferguson S: An education program on acquired immunodeficiency syndrome for patients with mental illness. Am J Occup Ther 49:359–361, 1995

Schneier FR, Siris SG: A review of psychoactive substance use and abuse in schizophrenia: patterns of drug choice. J Nerv Ment Dis 175:641–652, 1987

Seeman MV, Lang M, Rector N: Chronic schizophrenia: a risk factor for HIV? Can J Psychiatry 35:765–768, 1990

Silberstein C, Galanter M, Marmor M, et al: HIV-1 among inner city dually diagnosed patients. Am J Drug Alcohol Abuse 20:101–113, 1994

Sladyk K: Teaching safe sex practices to psychiatric patients. Am J Occup Ther 44:284–286, 1990

Stefan MD, Catalan J: Psychiatric patients and HIV infection: a new population at risk? Br J Psychiatry 167:721–727, 1995

Steiner J, Lussier R, Rosenblatt W: Knowledge about and risk factors for AIDS in a day hospital population. Hosp Community Psychiatry 43:734–735, 1992

Stewart DL, Zuckerman CJ, Ingle JM: HIV seroprevalence in a chronically mentally ill population. J Natl Med Assoc 86:519–523, 1994

Stiffman AR, Dore P, Earls F, et al: The influence of mental health problems on AIDS-related risk behaviors in young adults. J Nerv Ment Dis 180:314–320, 1992

Sullivan G, Koegal P, Kanouse D, et al: HIV and people with serious mental illness: the public sector's role in reducing HIV risk and improving care. Psychiatr Serv 50:648–652, 1999

Susser E, Valencia E, Conover S: Prevalence of HIV infection among psychiatric patients in a New York City men's shelter. Am J Public Health 83:568–570, 1993

Susser E, Valencia E, Miller M, et al: Sexual behavior of homeless mentally ill men at risk for HIV. Am J Psychiatry 152:583–587, 1995

Tate FB, Longo DA: HIV/AIDS prevention: a model for educating the inpatient psychiatric population. AIDS Patient Care STDS 14:325–331, 2000

Trixler M, Tenyi T: Antipsychotic use in pregnancy: what are the best treatment options? Drug Saf 16:403–410, 1997

Tynes LL, Sautter FJ, McDermott BE: Risk of HIV infection in the homeless and chronically mentally ill. South Med J 86:276–281, 1993

Volavka J, Convit A, Czobor P, et al: HIV seroprevalence and risk behaviors in psychiatric inpatients. Psychiatry Res 39:109–114, 1991

Volavka J, Convit A, O'Donnell J, et al: Assessment of risk behaviors for HIV infection among psychiatric inpatients. Hosp Community Psychiatry 43:482–485, 1992

Waldo MC, Roath M, Levine W, et al: A model program to teach parenting skills to schizophrenic mothers. Hosp Community Psychiatry 38:1110–1112, 1987

Walker A, Rosenberg M, Balaban-Gil K: Neurodevelopmental and neurobehavioral sequelae of selected substances of abuse and psychiatric medications in utero. Child Adolesc Clin North Am 8:845–867, 1999

Walkup J, Satriano J, Hansell S, et al: Practices related to HIV risk assessment in general hospital psychiatric units in New York State. Psychiatr Serv 49:529–530, 1998

Walkup J, McAlpine DD, Olfson M, et al: Recent HIV testing among general hospital inpatients with schizophrenia: findings from four New York City sites. Psychiatr Z 71:177–193, 2000

Wisner KL, Perel JM, Findling RL: Antidepressant treatment during breast-feeding. Am J Psychiatry 153:1132–1137, 1996

Wisner KL, Gelenberg AJ, Leonard H, et al: Pharmacologic treatment of depression during pregnancy. JAMA 282:1264–1269, 1999

Work Group on HIV/AIDS: Practice guidelines for the treatment of patients with HIV/AIDS. Am J Psychiatry 157:1–62, 2000

PART II

Psychiatric Disorders

3

Affective, Anxiety, and Somatoform Disorders and Dementia

INTRODUCTION

Depression, anxiety disorders, and somatoform disorders occupy a unique position in the interface between psychiatric illnesses and medical problems. Although many of the illnesses reviewed in this book have prominent, direct medical complications (for example, anorexia nervosa, bulimia nervosa, factitious disorder, and alcohol dependence), such associations are less clear for the illnesses discussed in this chapter. Still, some medical complications do occur in individuals with these illnesses, and there appear to be unique, complex causal links between depression and anxiety disorders and heart disease and hypertension.

In this chapter the link between anxiety disorders, depression, and medical illness will be reviewed, and the evidence connecting depression and anxiety symptoms to cardiac disease and hypertension will be examined. The potential medical complications of somatoform disorders will be reviewed using somatization disorder and hypochondriasis as examples, and suggestions for managing somatoform illnesses in conjunction with primary care providers will also be offered. Finally, several common medical complications of dementia will be examined.

DEPRESSION AND ANXIETY DISORDERS IN MEDICAL ILLNESS

Depression and anxiety disorders are known to be fairly common complications of a wide variety of medical conditions and appear to have an impact on the outcome of numerous illnesses. In this section we will briefly survey the literature on the occurrence of depression and anxiety in the context of medical illness and then examine the effect of these disorders on medical outcome.

Depression and Anxiety in Patients With Medical Illness

Table 3–1 summarizes several representative studies examining the frequency with which depression and anxiety occur in the medically ill. As the table shows, there is ample evidence indicating that depression and anxiety disorders appear to be more common in the medically ill than in the population at large. These increased rates range from modest elevations (for example, in coronary vascular disease) to reports of marked elevations (such as those found in some studies examining stroke).

Table 3–1. Rates of major depression in medical illness

Author	Medical illness	Prevalence, %
Popkin et al. 1988	Diabetes mellitus	24
Schleifer et al. 1989	Myocardial infarction	18
Starkstein 1989	Parkinson's disease	37
Kathol 1990	Various cancers	38
Robinson et al. 1984	Stroke	34
Eastwood et al. 1989	Stroke	50

To put these studies in perspective it is important to note that many of them examined patients over a relatively short time span: for example, the studies diagnosing depression following stroke have followed patients for no more than 3 years following stroke, and usually much closer to the time of their stroke. Thus, whereas the frequently cited population rates (from the Epidemiologic Catchment Area study, Weissman et al. 1988; or the National Comorbidity Survey, Blazer et al. 1994) present lifetime prevalence rates, many studies of the medically ill actually present prevalence rates over a very short timeframe of months or years following the medical diagnosis. Therefore, while the prevalence rates in these persons are higher than population prevalence rates, incidence rates appear to be even more elevated in comparison with population incidence rates. However, the high incidence of psychiatric illnesses in medical patients does not address the possible etiologic role of depression or anxiety in causing or exacerbating the medical illnesses.

An additional consideration in understanding depression as it occurs in the medically ill is the concept of demoralization. As described by

Slavney (1999), demoralization can represent a normal response to some situations and is thus distinct from both depression and adjustment disorder. As Slavney points out, the cornerstone of treatment in this situation is the approach taken by the physician in charge of the patient's care. In particular, being able to articulate an optimistic, well-thought-out treatment plan can be quite helpful. A major role for the psychiatrist in such a situation is to assist in accurately differentiating demoralization from depression or adjustment disorder.

Impact of Depression and Anxiety on the Course of Medical Illness

A major issue in the convergence of anxiety disorders and depression with medical illness is the impact of the psychiatric illness on medical outcome. Much as with the evidence on comorbidity noted above, studies examining several medical illnesses consistently suggest increased morbidity or mortality in depressed or anxious patients in comparison with nondepressed, nonanxious control subjects or other comparison groups.

Among the best studied of these relationships is the affect of depression on mortality in patients with cardiovascular disease. For example, Frasure-Smith et al. (1993, 1995) showed that depression is a powerful predictor of mortality at follow-up among post–myocardial infarction patients, conferring an increase in relative risk of around sixfold both at 6- and 18-month follow-up. More recent work has expanded this finding, with evidence for elevated cardiovascular mortality in depressed individuals in the community (Schulz et al. 2000) and in individuals with unstable angina (Lespérance et al. 2000).

The direct causal mechanism for this relationship is uncertain. Recent work in this area has focused in part on serotonin-mediated alterations of platelet function (Biegon et al. 1987; Laghrissi-Thode et al. 1997; Musselman et al. 1996, 1998). Changes in platelet serotonin receptor activity occurring in depression might increase the likelihood of platelet aggregation and clotting, and one recent study has demonstrated that paroxetine treatment significantly decreased markers of platelet activation such as β-thromboglobulin and platelet factor 4 (Pollock et al. 2000). A second hypothesized mechanism involves heart rate variability, which when diminished has been associated with cardiac sudden death. Such diminished heart rate variability has been found in depression (Carney et al. 1995; Rechlin et al. 1994).

Similar evidence exists documenting the adverse impact of depression on rehabilitation and functional outcome, and perhaps mortality, in stroke patients (Feibel and Springer 1982; Mayo et al. 1991; Parikh et al. 1990) as well as hip-fracture patients (Mossey et al. 1989, 1990). Depression has also been linked to worsened glycemic control in people with Type I diabetes (Eaton et al. 1992). It seems highly plausible that this link would lead to higher morbidity and mortality, although this link has not yet been definitively proven.

Depression and Anxiety as Risk Factors for Developing Physical Illness

Another area of interest in the interface between mood and anxiety disorders and medical illness is the possibility that medical illnesses could be directly caused by a preexisting mood or anxiety disorder. Such a link would fundamentally alter our understanding of anxiety disorders and depression, further emphasizing the need for early detection and treatment as an exercise in prevention.

Until recently, a causal link between depression and anxiety and the development of physical illness has been unproven; however, recent research suggests anxiety and depression may lead to the development of hypertension. Many of the early studies in this area failed to find a link between the development of hypertension and anxiety (Jenkins et al. 1983; Kahn et al. 1972; Russek et al. 1990; Sparrow et al. 1982) or depression (Goldberg et al. 1980). Several recent studies, however, have found such a link for anxiety alone (Markovitz et al. 1991, 1993) or for both depression and anxiety (Jonas et al. 1997). Perhaps of most interest is the recent study by Jonas et al. (1997). This was one of the largest studies in this area, examining nearly 3,000 subjects over a follow-up period ranging from 7 to 16 years. Standardized measures of both anxiety and depression were used. High levels of anxiety and depression symptoms at initial assessment were each predictive of new-onset hypertension by the end of the follow-up period.

A subsequent, similar finding has been described in the Johns Hopkins Precursors Study (Ford et al. 1998). This long-term, large (1,190 subjects) study was designed to examine risk factors for the development of coronary artery disease. At 40-year follow-up, subjects who had experienced clinical depression had higher risks of also having developed both coronary artery disease (relative risk [RR], 2.12; 95% confidence interval [CI], 1.24–3.63) and myocardial infarction (RR, 2.12; 95% CI, 1.11–4.06).

These studies represent the first clear links between the presence of a mood or anxiety disorder and the subsequent development of a medical complication. Presumably, successful treatment of the mood or anxiety disorder would ameliorate the risk of subsequent hypertension or coronary artery disease. This, however, is unproven and actually may be very difficult to prove. One reason, for example, is that strongly convincing evidence of the link between anxiety disorders, depression, and hypertension was shown only in a large sample of subjects followed for, on average, a decade. Randomization to years of participation in treated and untreated control groups would be ethically unacceptable; even if this were possible, very large sample sizes would be required. Thus, on the basis of available evidence, it seems reasonable to hypothesize that identifying and treating anxiety and mood disorders may diminish the risk for development of hypertension and coronary artery disease over the long term, although this will be difficult or impossible to prove.

Physiological Dysfunction in Depression

Studies examining the pathophysiology of major depression (and to a lesser extent, anxiety disorders) in the past several decades have delineated biochemical and/or physiological dysfunction in several physiologic systems, both within and outside the central nervous system. Many of these disruptions of normal function appear to involve systems not directly linked to central nervous system function, for example, alterations of immune function. One cautionary note: the clinical or pathophysiological significance of the disruptions of the functions described below remains largely undefined.

One area of intense interest has been the impact of depression on immune system function. Numerous parameters of immune function are altered in depression. Mitogen-stimulated lymphocyte proliferation is blunted (Kronfol and House 1989; O'Neill and Leonard 1990). Neutrophil phagocytic activity is diminished, although monocyte phagocytic activity may be increased (McAdams and Leonard 1993). Markers of humoral immunity are consistently elevated. A wide variety of acute-phase reactions are elevated, including immunoglobulins M and A, complement components C3 and C4, and numerous pro-inflammatory cytokines (Healy et al. 1991; Kronfol and House 1989; Maes et al. 1991, 1992a, 1992b).

A second area of interest has been the long-term effects of hypercortisolemia due to depression, anxiety, or stress. There are at least two potential detrimental effects of hypercortisolemia. The first, which has been the subject of substantial research interest, is its effect on cognitive function. Animal research has demonstrated a potential link between hypercortisolemia and hippocampal cell loss (Sapolsky et al. 1985; Squire 1992). On the basis of this evidence in conjunction with previous classic findings of hypercortisolemia occurring in depression (Carroll 1982), a number of investigators have looked for a relationship between markers of hypercortisolemia and cognitive function as well as changes in hippocampal volume. The results conflicted somewhat with certain studies linking hypercortisolemia and hippocampal volume (Axelson et al. 1993; Starkman et al. 1992;), but not with others (Coffey 1993). Similar conflicting evidence exists for measures of cognitive function (Newcomer et al. 1994; Starkman and Schteingart 1981; Wolkowitz et al. 1990). Of particular interest, one study examining the effects of chronic corticosteroid treatment for systemic illness has also found a decrement in memory function, which the investigators attributed to glucocorticoid usage (Keenan et al. 1996).

A second area of concern is the possibility that long-standing hypercortisolemia might predispose to bone mineral loss, osteoporosis, or other medical complications. Bone changes are a clearly identified side effect of the administration of corticosteroids. One might be particularly concerned about this problem given that the preponderance of patients with anxiety and mood disorders are women, who would be at higher risk for this complication. A variety of other adverse effects of exogenous corticosteroids have been described, but it is not known if endogenous hypercortisolemia has a similar effect.

Medical Management of Depression and Anxiety Disorders

The potential medical complications of depression and anxiety disorders are unique among those discussed in this book in that they are largely hypothetical, and for the most part specific medical interventions are not warranted. For example, specific surveillance for infection is not warranted in this population because clinical correlates of the immune dysfunction seen in these patient groups have not been identified. The one recommendation that might be made is to be sure to strongly encourage routine health care maintenance, specifically including blood pressure determination for anxious and depressed patients, given evidence now linking those illnesses and hypertension.

SOMATOFORM DISORDERS

The management of medical symptoms and medical complications associated with somatization disorder and hypochondriasis presents a challenge similar to that seen in factitious illness (see Chapter 5). These patients typically have a difficult relationship with the health care system.

Commonly they are high utilizers of emergent, urgent, and routine health care, presenting with what are widely appreciated to be "functional" physical complaints (Barsky et al. 1986). In this section, we will briefly review the challenges of caring for patients with somatoform disorders within the medical care system and discuss appropriate medical management.

Challenge for Primary Care Providers

Primary care providers have difficulty treating patients with somatoform disorders and often feel like they would prefer to treat "real" patients. They can become frustrated and at times angry with the patient—and also, at times, with the psychiatrist, whom they may come to believe "can't do anything about this patient" (Barsky et al. 1991). Thus, frustration with the process of caring for these patients represents the first major challenge in their comanagement by psychiatrists and primary care physicians.

A second challenge is that these patients are often undiagnosed. Surveys of primary care clinics have revealed that most patients who appear to meet criteria for somatization disorder and perhaps hypochondriasis are not diagnosed with a somatoform illness (Katon et al. 1992; Labott et al. 1995). One reason for this may be that the typical presenting symptoms are quite common among the nonsomatizing clinic population, for example, palpitations (Kroenke and Mangelsdorff 1989).

A third challenge is that not all of the symptoms experienced by patients with somatoform disorders are "functional." A major concern in the medical care of these patients is that the wide variety of reported symptoms is likely to lead eventually to diagnostic or therapeutic maneuvers that carry some iatrogenic risk. In this sense, these patients have some of the same potential medical complications as those with factitious illness (although the medical risks involved in inducing symptoms, as occurs in factitious illness, are not seen in somatization or hypochondriasis). Therein lies a particular challenge in the management of these patients: the physician involved must exercise appropriate restraint in conservatively managing many (perhaps most) symptoms with an approach of watchful waiting, while at the same time accurately distinguishing those symptoms that are "real" and require active intervention. Assisting in this process can be particularly difficult for psychiatrists, many of whom, by virtue of their training and practice experience, are somewhat less comfortable with this kind of evaluation. For example, the primary care practitioner accustomed to evaluating chest pain will usually be much more comfortable classifying chest pain as likely to be cardiac versus noncardiac, or "real" versus "functional."

A final challenge in the treatment of these patients is the experience of the patient not feeling understood, heard, or believed. Clinically, this often leads to a sense of anxiety or even desperation on the part of patients that their complaints will not be taken seriously or, in fact, will not even be heard at all (Ketterer and Buckholtz 1989). In response to this, the patient may barrage the primary care physician or psychiatrist with a list of complaints or concerns whose length greatly exceeds the amount of time available for a given clinical appointment. Such an experience is typically very frustrating for the physician with limited time available and a busy clinic schedule, leading to a temptation to schedule follow-up visits at the longest possible interval (Lin et al. 1991). This in turn reinforces the patient's need to have all the complaints heard in any given clinic visit because the next opportunity to do so is so far away. Thus, an escalating series of frustrations, on the part of both the caregivers and the patient, can occur.

Medical Management of Somatoform Disorders

One useful approach to the management of patients with somatoform disorders involves consistent collaboration between the psychiatrist and primary care provider (Smith 1988). Often the most important role for the psychiatrist is to assist in making or confirming the initial diagnosis and carefully assessing for (and treating) any associated comorbid conditions such as mood disorders, anxiety disorders, or substance use disorders. Medical management of these patients involves the routine health care maintenance employed by the primary care physician, with a few differences:

- It generally works best for these individuals to see a physician who is comfortable with, and perhaps even enjoys, the challenges of the somatizing patient.
- Such a physician ideally is comfortable trying to balance the appropriate use of aggressive diagnostic and therapeutic modalities with large doses of watchful waiting.
- It is usually advisable to schedule the patient for frequent visits even if there is no acute medical problem. Such an approach has several advantages. These include gradual reassurance of the patient that all concerns will be heard; the possibility of frequent reassessment, which may help the physician feel more comfortable about adopting a conservative management strategy; shorter individual clinic visits; and a decrease in "doctor shopping" by the patient.

An additional treatment approach that can be considered for patients with somatoform disorders involves the use of cognitive behavioral strategies. In many respects, this treatment is similar to those employed in other forms of cognitive behavioral therapy, but the focus is on the patient's cognitions about physical symptoms and sensations (Sharpe et al. 1992). In particular, a patient's interpretation of physical sensations as symptoms of illness is addressed, and potential factors that can serve to increase symptoms (such as some aspects of seeking medical help, as well as emotional distress) are identified.

DEMENTIA AND MENTAL DISORDERS DUE TO GENERAL MEDICAL CONDITIONS

Patients with dementia or mental disorders due to medical conditions are at high risk for a wide variety of medical complications. Several of these are highlighted in the following sections.

Urinary Incontinence

Urinary incontinence represents an important medical complication of dementia. Previous studies have reported incontinence rates for patients with dementia in various settings ranging from 11% to 90% (Skelly and Flint 1995). In contrast to rates in the general population, where incontinence is more common in women than men, in most of these reports the rates are higher in men than in women. A variety of risk factors for the occurrence of incontinence in dementia are listed in Table 3–2. Urinary incontinence can present in several fundamental ways in dementia. First, it can be a marker of a new or short-term problem, such as delirium or urinary tract infection. Second, it can represent the manifestation of a more long-term condition such as prostatic disease. Third, it can occur as a result of certain medications.

The initial management of urinary incontinence involves an evaluation to reveal the specific cause. The most appropriate starting place is a thorough history obtained both from the patient and from staff or family members familiar with the patient. A careful physical examination, including rectal and pelvic examination, is the appropriate next step. Limited laboratory evaluation is also required, including serum blood urea nitrogen, urinalysis to rule out urinary tract infection, and creatinine to examine kidney function. Measurement of post-voiding bladder residual volume by bladder catheterization after spontaneous voiding is used to assess for urine retention, with post-void residual volumes of 200 mL or more indicating urine retention (Urinary Incontinence Guideline Panel 1992). Careful attention should be paid to the medications the patient is receiving. Such a review should include careful scrutiny for drugs that

Table 3–2. Risk factors for urinary incontinence in dementia

Immobilization
Delirium
Prostatic surgery
Benign prostatic hypertrophy
Detrusor hyperactivity
Urinary tract infection
Antispasmodic/anticholinergic medications, e.g., bethanechol chloride, methacholine chloride, propantheline bromide, tricyclic antidepressants, oxybutynin chloride
Diuretic medications, e.g., hydrochlorothiazide, metolazone, furosemide, torsemide, spironolactone, triamterene
Antipsychotic medications

would increase urine volume such as diuretics; drugs that would prevent adequate bladder emptying such as anticholinergic drugs; and a variety of drugs that would serve to limit mobility and access to toileting, including antipsychotics and benzodiazepines.

At times, the definitive treatment of incontinence involves merely removing the offending drug or treating the underlying medical problem. Frequently, however, more involved measures are required. Options available for the treatment of incontinence are listed in Table 3–3. Some of the options listed may be useful for the majority of patients; these include the use of behavioral programs for frequent voiding and environmental interventions to eliminate physical barriers to toilet use (Hu et al. 1989; Schnelle 1990; Urinary Incontinence Guideline Panel 1992). Others are clearly more specific and determined by underlying causes of incontinence, for example, surgery or pharmacotherapy (Wein 1990). Pharmacotherapeutic strategies have primarily involved antispasmodic or anticholinergic agents. Two caveats are important to note in this regard, however. First, the use of anticholinergic agents in cognitively impaired individuals is problematic. There is evidence that anticholinergic agents such as scopolamine can adversely affect cognitive function, and it appears that individuals with dementia are particularly sensitive to these effects (Huff et al. 1988; Sunderland et al. 1985). Second, although these agents have been fairly effective in many trials, this has been much less true in cognitively impaired individuals (Skelly and Flint 1995).

Malnutrition

Previous studies have reported a relatively high frequency of malnutrition in older adults who are hospitalized (Gray 1989; Gray and Gray 1989;

Table 3–3. Treatment approaches for urinary incontinence

Behavioral toileting programs
Environmental interventions, e.g., removal of mobility barriers, modification of clothing for ease of toileting
Pharmacotherapy with antispasmodics, e.g., oxybutynin chloride, bethanechol chloride, propantheline chloride, methacholine chloride
Intermittent or chronic catheterization
Surgery, e.g., bladder neck reception, external sphincterotomy

Morley et al. 1988). Generally, however, this clinical problem receives little attention, both in the medically ill and in patients with dementia. This is an unfortunate oversight, because the presence of malnutrition appears to represent an important negative predictor in dementia. A recent study documented that the relative mortality risk associated with malnutrition in dementia was 1.31 (95% CI, 1.23–1.39); this risk was similar in magnitude to the risk conferred by cardiovascular disease or diabetes mellitus (Gambassi et al. 1999). Some of the potential causes of malnutrition in this group are listed in Table 3–4.

There are probably numerous reasons that many of these problems are commonly overlooked. Difficulties with eating as well as the occurrence of weight loss are seen as "normal" in older patients. Hospital personnel or nursing home staff rarely have experience assessing and understanding difficulties with swallowing, the adverse impact of edentulousness, and behaviors such as food hoarding. Also, especially in psychiatric settings, input from dietitians is often not available. Finally, in the hospitalized or institutionalized individual with a host of medical and behavioral problems, eating, although vital, is easy to overlook in favor of more acute problems.

Table 3–4. Causes of malnutrition in patients with dementia

Depression
Anorexia
Dysphagia
Hoarding food in the mouth
Eating apraxia
Food refusal
Food leaking from the mouth
Occult malignancy
Xerostomia
Helicobacter pylori infection
Impaired sense of smell

The initial management of malnutrition in patients with dementia involves careful review of recent weight history. Obviously, low weight and/or weight loss are major signs of malnutrition. Associated laboratory evidence, including measurement of serum transferrin and albumin, may be useful, and at times, so may markers of short-term starvation states such as elevated beta-hydroxybutyrate.

The patient should be evaluated to determine the underlying cause of the malnutrition. The medical workup should address the possibility of occult malignancy or gastritis caused by *Helicobacter pylori* infection. Problems such as depression should be detected in the initial psychiatric evaluation, but the presence of malnutrition may provide a trigger for re-evaluation. Careful assessment of the patient's dentition (whether natural or artificial) is appropriate. Motoric ability to feed oneself and the ability to masticate and swallow food also must be evaluated. Consultation with occupational and/or speech therapists and, at times, radiologic examination can help with this assessment, but often careful history from nursing home personnel, hospital personnel, or family will go a long way toward understanding these contributing factors. Finally, a period of careful monitoring of dietary intake may help to uncover the type and extent of protein/calorie malnutrition. In particular, assessment of intake pattern may be helpful, because eating compliance may be substantially better with one meal than with the others (Stahelin et al. 1983). If so, it may be helpful to focus on the meal or meals that the patient most successfully eats.

A dietitian is typically central in the management of malnutrition and restoration of body weight, strength, and good nutrition. The provision of adequate nutrition involves first identifying an adequate number of calories for the patient. The dietician can then assist the patient in choosing specific foods and diets to meet nutritional needs. For example, a puréed diet may be helpful for some individuals, while for others, such textures may contribute to poor food intake. Similarly, if sense of smell is impaired, more intensely flavorful foods may be useful (Marcus and Berry 1998). In addition to observing weight, it may be useful to follow serum albumin and transferrin as additional markers of nutritional status.

Falls

Falling represents a major medical problem in the age group at greatest risk for dementia, the geriatric population. Dementia or other cognitive impairment is in and of itself a significant risk factor for falls; so too are the use of psychiatric medications and a number of medical and sensory problems commonly found in patients with dementia. Falling, a broad clinical phenomenon with a variety of possible causes, has been classically defined as "an unplanned slip to the floor" with or without injury (Lawrence and Maher 1992). Within this broad category are a variety of potential etiologies, as shown in Table 3–5. These can be broken out broadly into falls due to a specific medical process or symptom (stroke, arrhythmia, orthostasis, and other causes of syncope) and falls related to issues specific to the environment or the patient. The most pertinent etiologies for this chapter are dementia and other cognitive impairments.

The most important step in managing a patient who has fallen is an initial assessment of any trauma sustained in the fall and assessment for potential etiologies of falling. A thorough physical and neurological examination, assessment of mental status, and an electrocardiogram are useful initial steps in assessing patients when the clinical picture or examination is strongly suggestive of cerebral vascular accident. Immediate evaluation in an emergency department is appropriate. In this instance, and also in patients with loss of consciousness or apparent head trauma (especially in those with a risk factor for intracranial bleeding, such as anticoagulant therapy), a central nervous system imaging study is probably also appropriate. A major focus of the initial evaluation is to look for evidence of trauma including bone fractures (especially of the hip), joint dislocation, or closed head injury.

A critically important part of the management of the patient who falls is secondary prevention. Obviously attention should be paid to any significant medical problems that have an impact on this risk, such as orthostasis, dehydration, and sedation from long-acting benzodiazepines or neuroleptics or other sedating medications. Environmental modifications, including the provision of adequate lighting, the elimination of loose rugs, and the avoidance of slippery shoes, can diminish risk. Also, sensory problems including changes in vision should be assessed. Occupational and/or physical therapy assessments may be useful in evaluating balance, ability to transfer, and walking.

Table 3–5. Factors associated with falling

Increasing age
Receiving multiple medications
Orthostatic hypotension
Sensory deficits
Mobility impairments
Cardiovascular disease
Cerebrovascular disease
Other neurologic diseases

SUMMARY

Depression and anxiety occur more frequently in patients with certain medical illnesses, and there is evidence that they may be associated with worse medical outcomes. A number of physiological systems do show evidence of dysfunction in anxiety and depression, although the clinical significance of this finding is as yet undetermined. Depression and anxiety appear to represent important risk factors for developing hypertension and coronary artery disease. Awareness of this by psychiatrists may help prevent medical complications.

Somatization disorder can be particularly challenging for both psychiatrist and primary care provider. Complications of therapeutic and diagnostic procedures for somatized symptoms represent the major medical morbidity and mortality of this illness. Careful attention to diagnosis, coordination of care between the psychiatrist and a primary care provider familiar with management of these patients, and frequent primary care visits represent a useful strategy in managing these individuals.

Several common medical complications may occur in patients with dementia, delirium, and mental disorders due to general medical conditions. Urinary incontinence can cause significant discomfort and represents a major burden for caregivers. Falls and malnutrition each can increase the risk for mortality. A variety of often simple interventions can address each of these problems.

REFERENCES

Axelson DA, Doraiswamy PM, McDonald WM, et al: Hypercortisolemia and hippocampal changes in depression. Psychiatry Res 47:163–173, 1993

Barsky AJ, Wyshak G, Klerman GL: Medical and psychiatric determinants of outpatient medical utilization. Med Care 24:548–560, 1986

Barsky AJ, Wyshak G, Latham KS: Hypochondriacal patients, their physicians, and their medical care. J Gen Intern Med 6:413–419, 1991

Biegon A, Weizman A, Karp L, et al: Serotonin 5-HT2 receptor binding on blood platelets: a peripheral marker for depression? Life Sci 41:2485–2492, 1987

Blazer DG, Kessler RC, McGonagle KA, et al: The prevalence and distribution of major depression in a national community sample: the National Comorbidity Survey. Am J Psychiatry 151:979–986, 1994

Carney RM, Saunders RD, Freedland KE, et al: Association of depression with reduced heart rate variability in coronary artery disease. Am J Cardiol 76:562–564, 1995

Carroll BJ: The dexamethasone suppression test for melancholia. Br J Psychiatry 140:292–304, 1982

Coffey CE, Wilkinson WC, Weiner R: The dexamethasone suppression test and quantitative cerebral anatomy in depression. Biol Psychiatry 33:442–449, 1993

Eastwood MR, Rifat SL, Nobbs H, et al: Mood disorder following cerebrovascular accident. Br J Psychiatry 154:195–200, 1989

Eaton WW, Mengel M, Mengel L, et al: Psychosocial and psychopathologic influences on management and control of insulin-dependent diabetes. Int J Psychiatry Med 22:105–117, 1992

Feibel JH, Springer CJ: Depression and failure to resume social activities after stroke. Arch Phys Med Rehabil 63:276–278, 1982

Ford DE, Mead LA, Chany PP, et al: Depression is a risk factor for coronary artery disease in men. Arch Intern Med 158:1422–1426, 1998

Frasure-Smith N, Lespérance F, Talajic M: Depression following myocardial infarction: impact on 6-month survival. JAMA 270:1819–1825, 1993

Frasure-Smith N, Lespérance F, Talajic M: Depression and 18-month prognosis after myocardial infarction. Circulation 91:999–1005, 1995

Gambassi G, Landi F, Lapane KL, et al: Predictors of mortality in patients with Alzheimer's disease living in nursing homes. J Neurol Neurosurg Psychiatry 67:59–65, 1999

Goldberg EL, Comstock GW, Graves CG: Psychological factors and blood pressure. Psychol Med 10:243–255, 1980

Gray GE: Nutrition and dementia. J Am Diet Assoc 89:1795–1802, 1989

Gray GE, Gray LK: Nutritional aspects of psychiatric disorders. J Am Diet Assoc 89:1492–1498, 1989

Healy D, Calvin J, Whitehouse AM, et al: Alpha-1-acid glycoprotein in major depressive and eating disorders. J Affect Disord 2:13–20, 1991

Hu TW, Igou JF, Kaltreider L, et al: A clinical trial of a behavioral therapy to reduce urinary incontinence in nursing homes. JAMA 261:2656–2662, 1989

Huff FJ, Mickel SF, Corkin S, et al: Cognitive functions affected by scopolamine in Alzheimer's disease and normal aging. Drug Development Research 12:271–278, 1988

Jenkins CD, Somervell PD, Hames CG: Does blood pressure usually rise with age? Or with stress? J Human Stress 9:4–12, 1983

Jonas BS, Franks P, Ingram DD: Are symptoms of anxiety and depression risk factors for hypertension? Arch Fam Med 6:43–49, 1997

Kahn HA, Medalie JH, Neufeld HN, et al: The incidence of hypertension and associated factors: the Israel Ischemic Heart Disease Study. Am Heart J 84:171–182. 1972

Kathol RG, Mutgi A, Williams J, et al: Diagnosis of major depression in cancer patients according to four sets of criteria. Am J Psychiatry 1990 147:1021–1024

Katon W, Kleinman A, Rosen G: Depression and somatization. Am J Med 72:127–135, 1982

Keenan PA, Jacobson MW, Soleymani RM, et al: The effect on memory of chronic prednisone treatment in patients with systemic disease. Neurology 47:1396–1402, 1996

Ketterer MW, Buckholtz CD: Somatization disorder. J Am Osteopath Assoc 89:489–499, 1989

Kroenke K, Mangelsdorff AD: Common symptoms in ambulatory care: incidence, evaluation, therapy, and outcome. Am J Med 86:262–266, 1989

Kronfol Z, House JD: Lymphocyte mitogenesis, immunoglobin and complement levels in depressed patients and normal controls. Acta Psychiatr Scand 80:142–147, 1989

Labott SM, Preisman RC, Popovich J, et al: Health care utilization of somatizing patients in a pulmonary subspecialty clinic. Psychosomatics 36:122–128, 1995

Laghrissi-Thode F, Finkel MS, Johnson PC, et al: Elevated platelet factor 4 and β-thromboglobulin plasma levels in depressed patients with ischemic heart disease. Biol Psychiatry 42:290–295, 1997

Lawrence J, Maher P: An interdisciplinary falls consult team: a collaborative approach to patient falls. J Nurs Care 6:21–29, 1992

Lespérance F, Frasure-Smith N, Juneau M, et al: Depression and 1-year prognosis in unstable angina. Arch Intern Med 160:1354–1360, 2000

Lin EHB, Katon W, VonKorff M, et al: Frustrating patients. J Gen Intern Med 6:241–246, 1991

Maes M, Bosmans E, Suy E, et al: Depression-related disturbances in mitogen-induced lymphocyte responses and interleukin-1b and soluble interleukin-2-receptor production. Acta Psychiatr Scand 84:379–386, 1991

Maes M, Scharpe S, van Grottel L, et al: Higher alpha-1-antitrypsin, haptoglobin, ceruloplasmin and lower retinol binding protein plasma levels during depression: further evidence for the existence of an acute phase response. J Affect Disord 24:183–192, 1992a

Maes M, Planken VD, Stevens WJ, et al: Leukocytosis, monocytosis and neutrophilia: hallmarks of severe depression. J Psychiatr Res 26:125–134, 1992b

Marcus EL, Berry EM: Refusal to eat in the elderly. Nutr Rev 56:163–171, 1998

Markovitz JH, Matthews KA, Wing RR, et al: Psychological, biological and health behavior predictors of blood pressure changes in middle-aged women. J Hypertens 9:399–406, 1991

Markovitz HJ, Matthews KA, Kannel WB, et al: Psychological predictors of hypertension in the Framingham Study: is there tension in hypertension? JAMA 270:2439–2443, 1993

Mayo NE, Korner-Bitensky NA, Becker R: Recovery time of independent function post-stroke. Am J Phys Med Rehabil 70:5–12, 1991

McAdams C, Leonard BE: Neutrophil and monocyte phagocytosis in depressed patients. Prog Neuropsychopharmacol 17:971–984, 1993

Morley JE, Mooradian AD, Silver AJ: Nutrition in the elderly. Ann Intern Med 109:890–904, 1988

Mossey JM, Mutran E, Knott K, et al: Determinants of recovery 12 months after hip fracture: the importance of psychosocial factors. Am J Public Health 79:279–286, 1989

Mossey JM, Knott K, Craik R: The effects of persistent depressive symptoms on hip fracture recovery. J Gerontol 45:M163–M168, 1990

Musselman DL, Tomer A, Manatungo AK, et al: Exaggerated platelet reactivity in major depression. Am J Psychiatry 153:1313–1317, 1996

Musselman DL, Evans DL, Nemeroff CB: The relationship of depression to cardiovascular disease: epidemiology, biology and treatment. Arch Gen Psychiatry 55:580–592, 1998

Newcomer JW, Craft S, Hershey T, et al: Glucocorticoid-induced impairment in explicit memory performance in adult humans. J Neurosci 14:2047–2053, 1994

O'Neill B, Leonard BE: Abnormal zymosan-induced neutrophil chemiluminescence as a marker of depression. J Affect Disord 19:265–272, 1990

Parikh RM Robinson RG, Lipsey JR, et al: The impact of poststroke depression on recovery in activities of daily living over a 2-year follow-up. Arch Neurol 47:786–789, 1990

Pollock BG, Laghrissi-Thode F, Wagner WR: Evaluation of platelet activation in depressed patients with ischemic heart disease after paroxetine or nortriptyline treatment. J Clin Psychopharmacol 20:137–140, 2000

Popkin MK, Callies AL, Lentz RD, et al: Prevalence of major depression, simple phobia, and other psychiatric disorders in patients with long-standing Type I diabetes mellitus. Arch Gen Psychiatry 45:64–68, 1988

Rechlin T, Weis M, Aspitzer A, et al: Are affective disorders associated with alterations of heart rate variability? J Affect Disord 32:271–275, 1994

Robinson RG, Starr LB, Price TR: A two year longitudinal study of mood disorders following stroke. Br J Psychiatry 144:256–262, 1984

Russek LG, King SH, Russek SJ, et al: The Harvard Mastery of Stress Study 35-year follow-up: prognostic significance of patterns of psychophysiological arousal and adaptation. Psychosom Med 52:271–285, 1990

Sapolsky RM, Krey LC, McEwen BS: Prolonged glucocorticoid exposure reduces hippocampal neuron number: implications for aging. J Neurosci 5:1222–1227, 1985

Schleifer SJ, Macari-Hinson MM, Coyle DA, et al: The nature and course of depression following myocardial infarction. Arch Intern Med 149:1785–1789, 1989

Schnelle JF: Treatment of urinary incontinence in nursing home patients by prompted voiding. J Am Geriatr Soc 38:356–360, 1990

Schulz R, Beach SR, Ives DG, et al: Association between depression and mortality in older adults. Arch Intern Med 160:1761–1768, 2000

Sharpe M, Peveler R, Mayou R: The psychological treatment of patients with functional somatic symptoms: a practical guide. J Psychosom Res 36:515–529, 1992

Skelly J, Flint AJ: Urinary incontinence associated with dementia. J Am Geriatr Soc 43:286–294, 1995

Slavney PR: Diagnosing demoralization in consultation psychiatry. Psychosomatics 40:325–329, 1999

Smith RC: Somatization in primary care. Clin Obstet Gynecol 31:902–914, 1988

Sparrow D, Garvey AJ, Rosener B, et al: Factors in predicting blood pressure change. Circulation 65:789–794, 1982

Squire LR: Memory and the hippocampus: a synthesis from findings with rats, monkeys, and humans. Psychol Rev 99:195–231, 1992

Stahelin HB, Hofer HO, Vogel M, et al: Energy and protein consumption in patients with senile dementia. Gerontology 29:145–148, 1983

Starkman MN, Schteingart DE: Neuropsychiatric manifestations of patients with Cushing's syndrome: relationship to cortisol and adrenocorticotropic hormone levels. Arch Intern Med 141:215–219, 1981

Starkman MN, Gebarski SS, Berent S: Hippocampal formation volume, memory dysfunction, and cortisol levels in patients with Cushing's syndrome. Biol Psychiatry 32: 756–765, 1992

Starkstein SE, Berthier ML, Bolduc PL, et al: Depression in patients with early versus late onset of Parkinson's disease. Neurology 39:1441–1445, 1989

Sunderland T, Tariot P, Murphy DL, et al: Scopolamine challenges in Alzheimer's disease. Psychopharmacology (Berl) 87:247–249, 1985

Urinary Incontinence Guideline Panel: Urinary Incontinence in Adults: Clinical Practice Guideline (AHCPR Pub. No. 92-0038). Rockville, MD, Agency for Health Care Policy and Research, U.S. Public Health Service, 1992

Wein AJ: Pharmacologic treatment of incontinence. J Am Geriatr Soc 38:317–325, 1990.

Weissman MM, Leaf PJ, Tischler GL, et al: Affective disorders in five United States communities. Psychol Med 18:141–153, 1988

Wolkowitz OM, Reus VI, Weingartner H, et al: Cognitive effects of corticosteroids. Am J Psychiatry 147:1297–1303, 1990

4

Schizophrenia and Other Psychotic Disorders

INTRODUCTION

It is not uncommon for patients with schizophrenia and other psychoses to develop medical problems (Lipper and Werman 1977; Vieweg et al. 1995). Some such problems may result directly from the patients' psychotic symptoms, such as foreign-body ingestion and self-mutilation, while others result from the development of common medical illnesses such as coronary artery disease and cancer (Adler and Griffith 1991; Babigian and Odoroff 1969; Baldwin 1979; Cutting 1980; Kampmeier 1977). It is worth noting that the prevalence of both types of problems may be different among patients with schizophrenia than among the general population.

In this chapter, we review several of these medical complications, cite their prevalence in this population wherever possible, and review the literature on clinical recognition of these problems (Hussar 1966). We then explore the physical and laboratory findings that may be useful in assessing these conditions and discuss their medical management. In addition to complications specifically associated with schizophrenia (self-injury and self-mutilation, foreign-body ingestion, polydipsia and water intoxication), we also discuss data on the prevalence of common medical conditions, such as coronary artery disease and cancer, in patients with schizophrenia, although the management of such disorders is beyond the scope of this chapter. Additionally, we review the challenges in diagnosing and treating medical illness in psychotic individuals, given their difficulties in communication and their frequent lack of insight into the nature of the problems they experience. Finally, we also touch on problems associated with pregnancy in patients with schizophrenia.

SELF-INJURY AND SELF-MUTILATION

The exact nature of medical problems resulting from self-induced injury depends on the site and severity of the injury and can range from modest skin lacerations that may require suturing to medical emergencies such as self-castration or self-enucleation.

The literatures on self-mutilation and self-injurious behavior overlap (Favazza 1989; Herpertz 1995; Langbehn and Pfohl 1993), but in general the available studies support the observation that self-injury can occur among various types of psychiatric patients and is not confined to patients with schizophrenia. However, self-injury in this group of patients is reported frequently enough to be of concern to the practicing clinician and to be of particular interest. Self-injury often focuses on certain parts of the body in this group of patients, usually the genitalia or the eyes.

Self-induced eye injury in patients with schizophrenia is frequently linked to a religious theme (Witherspoon et al. 1989), and often to a particular passage from the book of Matthew:

> If thy right eye offend thee, pluck it out and cast it from thee: for it is profitable for thee that only thy member should perish, not that thy whole body should be cast into hell; and if thy right hand offend thee, cut it off and cast it from thee: for it is profitable for thee that one of thy members should perish, and not that thy whole body be cast into hell. (Matt. 5:29–30)

Various types of eye damage can be seen in patients with schizophrenia, including aversion of the eyelid, scratching of the cornea and/or conjunctiva, and the introduction of infection, at times complicated by the development of periorbital abscess (Feldman 1988). However, the most extreme example is self-enucleation (Crowder et al. 1979; MacLean and Robertson 1976; Tobias et al. 1988). In 1994, Kennedy and Feldmann reviewed the literature in this area, finding a total of 41 cases in the psychiatric literature published between 1980 and 1993, and added 4 additional cases. The most frequent diagnosis among those who had damaged their own eyes was schizophrenia (55.6% of the cases), and the most common form of eye injury was self-enucleation (35.5%), with the most common mediating variable being religious preoccupation.

Another form of self-injury occurring in schizophrenia is genital self-mutilation (Blacker 1963; Young and Feinsilver 1986). It is worth noting that almost all of these cases have occurred in males. In a review, Martin and Gattaz (1991) found a total of 57 cases in the English-language literature as well as 5 in the German literature, and these authors added 2 more cases both involving self-castration. Most of the patients discussed in this review were psychotic, often diagnosed as having schizophrenia, and Martin and Gattaz (1991) drew renewed attention to the passage quoted above from the book of Matthew as being associated with this problem. Nakaya (1996) reviewed a total of 105 cases from the English-language literature, adding 5 new Japanese cases. The age range of those who engaged in genital self-mutilation was 17–72 years with a mean age of 36, and again the most common diagnosis was psychosis, often schizophrenia. Other risk factors included a history of self-mutilation, guilt feelings about sex, and sexual identity disturbance. The most common form of genital self-mutilation was complete transection of the penis, with or without autocastration.

Genital self-mutilation appears to be much rarer among psychotic women. Krasucki et al. (1995) reviewed two earlier reports of genital self-mutilation among women (a 20-year-old woman with schizophrenia who lacerated her cervix and vaginal vault by inserting foreign objects in response to command hallucinations and a 33-year-old woman who lacerated her labia in response to delusions that she had genital warts). They added the case of a woman who lacerated her labia, but the diagnosis in this case was unclear although the case report suggested a psychotic illness.

Other forms of mutilation appear to be less common, and include self-inflicted burns (Daniels et al. 1991), self-amputation of the ear (Alroe and Gunda 1995), autoextraction of teeth (Altom and DiAngelis 1989; Paterson et al. 1992), and tissue death in the distal phalanx of a finger secondary to chronic use of a rubber-band ligature (Birrer et al. 1993). Forms of self-mutilation also occur in odd combinations, including partial tongue removal combined with genital self-mutilation (Culliford 1987) or with self-enucleation (Garcia-Estrada 1988).

These complications range from the obvious (e.g., self-enucleation) to the obscure (e.g., the lesion is hidden and does not involve serious blood loss, and the patient does not report having injured himself). Although the number of case reports would suggest that self-injury is rare, there is also the possibility that such problems at times go overlooked.

Laboratory examination will be dictated by the nature and extent of the lesion and will usually require consultation (e.g., with surgery and/or urology in the case of genital mutilation, with ophthalmology in the case of eye self-injury). Emergency ophthalmologic consultation may be critical in preserving as much vision as possible in cases with partial enucleation.

Management will be dictated by the nature and severity of the injury and may necessitate emergency medical care in a well-staffed hospital emergency department, followed by aggressive medical or surgical care. Patients may require physical and/or chemical restraint, and a high priority must be placed on preventing the patient from engaging in further self-injury. Such patients may require constant observation for a protracted period of time (Shore et al. 1978). Given that a high percentage of patients who eventually progress to severe problems such as self-enucleation or transection of the penis have a history of more minor self-mutilation, efforts at self-injury that appear trivial must be regarded as possible precursors of further damage and must be taken seriously. Patients should be carefully questioned about religious preoccupations, religious delusions, and the presence or absence of command hallucinations (Hall et al. 1981). Treatment also involves aggressive pharmacotherapy of the underlying psychotic process.

The prognosis for patients who self-mutilate is difficult to predict without making certain assumptions regarding the type and severity of the injury. Transection of the penis and partial self-enucleation may to some extent be reversible, at least theoretically, but given the patient's frequent lack of insight into the necessity for rapid intervention and the attendant delays involved, such cases have not been documented in the literature. Therefore, in general the goal should be to minimize further damage and address the underlying psychotic illness.

WATER INTOXICATION

The syndrome variously described as polydipsia, hyponatremia syndrome, or water intoxication has been well documented among patients with schizophrenia for most of the past century. This complication is of considerable interest because it develops fairly commonly and can be associated with significant morbidity and mortality if not diagnosed and properly managed.

The incidence of this complication is not well established, at least partially owing to the fact that the severity of presentation may vary dramatically. One way of classifying cases is to stratify them into three stages, from mild to severe: 1) polydipsia; 2) polydipsia plus water intoxication (asymptomatic hyponatremia); and 3) physical complications of the intoxication and hyponatremia (de Leon et al. 1994). The prevalence of polydipsia has been reported to be approximately 20% in a chronic psychiatric population, with 5% progressing to water intoxication. In another prevalence study examining a state hospital population cross-sectionally, 42% were found to have polydipsia, with a rate of water intoxication of approximately 5% (de Leon et al. 1996). Significantly, almost all the prevalence data are on institutionalized populations, and the prevalence among outpatients is unknown.

The pathogenesis of this disorder is complicated, and the etiology may vary across patients. However, various clinical factors have been implicated, including the side effects of medication (e.g., use of anticholinergics for neuroleptic side effects inducing dry mouth), excessive water intake (boredom, abnormal thirst), a drive toward a sense of intoxication, and impaired excretory function, with, at times, inappropriate antidiuretic hormone secretion. It is worth noting that chronically mentally ill patients (even those not medicated with psychotropic drugs), when given a water load challenge, do evidence decreased cumulative urine output and have increased minimal urine osmolality (Emsley et al. 1989).

The complications of water intoxication may be life threatening. Hyponatremia syndrome in psychotic patients has been associated with evidence of brain structural abnormalities on computed tomography scanning (Emsley et al. 1995) and cognitive impairment on neurological testing (Emsley et al. 1993). Severe hyponatremia can result in permanent neurologic deficits and even death. Risk factors for the development of this complication, in addition to the diagnosis of schizophrenia, include smoking, chronicity of symptoms, and male gender (de Leon et al. 1994; Shutty 1996).

The clinical presentation can be highly variable but in addition to the polydipsia and polyuria, is often characterized by restlessness, diarrhea, nausea, and vomiting, with the subsequent development of tremor and muscle twitching, ataxia, and eventual progression to convulsions, stupor, and coma (Fleischhacker et al. 1987; Vieweg et al. 1994). The phenomenon has also been associated with rhabdomyolysis (Akasaki et al. 1993).

When supplying the pertinent history, most patients do not view their excess intake of fluids as problematic and will have no complaints. It is far more likely that family members or clinical staff will notice the excessive fluid intake, and in suspected cases information from caregivers regarding fluid intake should be obtained. Physical examination may reveal evidence of hypertonic reflexes, a clouded sensorium, and at times frank delirium. Often a brief period of observation as well as careful monitoring of weights over the course of a day will confirm the excessive water intake.

Laboratory assessment should focus on serum and urinary sodium and other electrolytes. Serum hyponatremia, at times severe, is the hallmark of the problem. Also, low serum and urine osmolalities are suggestive of excessive water intake. Many times the most useful information is obtained through intake and output records over a period of 8–12 hours to document both the polydipsia and the polyuria.

The medical management of such patients depends on the severity of the hyponatremia and the neurologic status. Among patients with polydipsia for whom the fluid intake has not yet resulted in critically low sodium, close monitoring of intake and output with emphasis on fluid restriction if necessary, as well as aggressive management of residual psychotic symptoms, appears to be indicated. It is of interest that the use of electrolyte-containing fluids such as Gatorade, available on an as-needed basis, does not appear to attenuate the development of this disorder (Goldman et al. 1994). For patients who have progressed to significant hyponatremia, more aggressive therapy may be necessary, in conjunction with consultation by an internist, neurologist, or other experienced specialist. In all suspected cases, a neurologic examination should be performed to detect possible unexplained changes in mental status or focal neurologic findings.

The literature on the treatment of this condition has been summarized recently by Vieweg (1994) and Vieweg et al. (1994). Treatment interventions are offered in Table 4–1. The early treatment interventions for this condition, which were described decades ago, centered on the use of supplemental sodium administration and fluid restriction. These approaches remain the cornerstones in the management of hyponatremia. The rapidity with which the hyponatremia develops will dictate the severity of symptoms. One patient may chronically have a serum sodium of 120 mm/dL and be asymptomatic, whereas another who acutely develops a comparable sodium concentration may have dramatic symptoms requiring urgent hospitalization.

Several drug therapy regimens have been suggested. The three drugs that have been used most commonly are lithium, demeclocycline, and phenytoin. Both lithium and demeclocycline counteract the renal action of arginine vasopressin and facilitate free water clearance. The mechanism through which phenytoin acts is unknown. Most of the available data on the utility of these compounds is based on case reports or small series of patients. Demeclocycline is usually administered in an oral dose of 300–400 mg three or four times daily. As reviewed by Vieweg (1994), treatment with this agent may not prove effective for 4–6 weeks, and therefore it is not uncommon for physicians to abandon trials of the agent prematurely. Lithium and phenytoin in standard therapeutic doses have also been reported to be useful adjuncts in the treatment of some patients, although the data are quite limited. Other agents that have been used include propranolol, angiotensin-converting enzyme inhibitors, and fluoxetine.

FOREIGN-BODY INGESTION

There is a large medical and surgical literature on foreign-body ingestion, much of it involving children. When focusing on this phenomenon

Table 4–1. Interventions for water intoxication

Serum sodium concentrations	Interventions
Sodium 125–130 mmol/mL and patient asymptomatic	Patient should be limited to less than 3 L of fluid intake per day. Also consider giving 4.5 g sodium chloride by mouth.
Sodium 120–125 mmol/mL and patient asymptomatic	Give 4.5 g sodium chloride by mouth, repeat in 2 hours. Restrict patient to area without access to water and monitor weight, with close, frequent follow-up required.
Sodium 115–120 mmol/mL and patient asymptomatic	Give 4.5 g sodium chloride by mouth and repeat dose hourly. Hospitalize patient, restrict to room, observe closely, and consult with internist.
Sodium < 115 mmol/mL and/or patient symptomatic (altered mental status, seizures, etc.)	Inpatient management by an internist is most appropriate. If patient develops seizures or becomes comatose, administer 3%–5% hypertonic saline IV over 2–3 hours, being careful not to raise serum sodium concentrations above 1–2 mmol/L/hour. Overly rapid correction of sodium can result in central pontine myelinolysis.

in adults, however, many of the case reports mention or suggest the presence of a psychosis, often schizophrenia. The reports that appear in the medical literature undoubtedly represent the more unusual cases, and it is difficult to generalize from these. Examples include a 46-year-old woman who was found to have both a screw and a nail in a main bronchus and an open safety pin in her gut (Jacob et al. 1990); a patient who was found to have 82 metallic objects in his gastrointestinal tract (Kikoler et al. 1992); and a patient who was found to have ingested 71 objects, including coins, metal wire, keys, and screws (Slovis et al. 1982). The reasons given by the patient for the ingestion are usually not mentioned, and it is clearly impossible to estimate the true prevalence of such problems.

Patients may or may not admit to such ingestions, and many cases undoubtedly never come to light. Relative to the diagnosis and treatment, the nature of the presumed ingested object or objects will dictate whether or not they will be visible on plain X ray (e.g., metallic) or require the introduction of a radio-opaque contrast substance to be detected (e.g., glass).

The reassuring finding is that 90% of ingested objects generally pass through the intestinal tract without the patient requiring surgery (Slovis et al. 1982), including such objects as open pins and glass. It may take objects 1–3 days to pass, however. Generally, surgery is indicated when the object fails to progress through the gastrointestinal tract or if there is evidence of obstruction, gastrointestinal bleeding, or perforation (O'Sullivan et al. 1996). Patients may practice variations on the theme of foreign-body ingestion, such as inserting foreign matter into the ear (Weiser et al. 1993).

CARDIOVASCULAR DISEASE AND OTHER COMMON MEDICAL ILLNESSES

Over the years, a fairly large literature has accumulated suggesting that patients with schizophrenia may develop certain medical illnesses at frequencies different from the prevalence of such disorders in the general population. Some of the findings in this area are only suggestive of differential rates, whereas others appear to be well established.

Relative to cancer, several reports suggest lower than expected rates for many malignancies in patients with schizophrenia (Katz et al. 1967; Massie 1989; Masterson and O'Shea 1984). Of particular note, the rate of lung cancer does not appear to be elevated despite the fact that rates of cigarette smoking are very high among patients with schizophrenia (Goff et al. 1992; Gopalaswamy and Morgan 1986; Hughes et al. 1986). The reasons for this apparent discrepancy are unclear.

Overall, mortality is clearly increased in schizophrenia, predominantly due to increased risk of suicide and accidents; however, several studies suggest that patients with schizophrenia may have increased mortality from infections and other "natural" diseases compared with the general population (Buda et al. 1988). Perhaps most striking are reports documenting low rates of asthma, hay fever, and, in particular, rheumatoid arthritis in this patient population, which may conceivably be attributable in part to the antihistaminic effects of many psychotropic drugs (Ehrentheil 1957; Osterberg 1978). Rates of cardiovascular disease may be similar to those in the general population, but, again, given the high prevalence of smoking and the documented relationship between smoking and cardiovascular disease, this may be interpreted as somewhat surprising (Vieweg et al. 1994). Other variables that might have an impact on this prevalence, including lack of exercise, would imply higher rates, yet such elevated rates have not been documented.

MANAGEMENT OF THE PREGNANT PATIENT WITH SCHIZOPHRENIA

Management of pregnancy in patients with schizophrenia can be quite problematic (Burgess 1980). Although the course of the psychosis during a pregnancy can be highly variable, not uncommonly psychiatric symptoms worsen in this population as opposed to those with other forms of psychopathology (Spielvogel and Wile 1986). Several issues need to be considered regarding this group of patients (Muqtadir et al. 1986; Spielvogel and Wile 1986). First are the legal implications involved. In most states, health care providers have a clear duty to protect an unborn child and are given the legal obligation to intervene if patients pose a threat to themselves or others. This necessitates a careful assessment of the patient's ability to adequately manage the welfare of her fetus. Not uncommonly, it involves a court order requiring the patient to follow through with prenatal care plans; the court may suggest or require hospitalization for severely psychotic individuals. The legal definition and requirements will vary by state, but careful consideration and assessment of these issues should be part of the early management of these cases, and the involvement of the psychiatrist is essential.

These patients can have a great deal of difficulty cooperating with even routine medical monitoring such as prenatal examinations and diagnostic testing. It is very useful to have a mental health care professional, often a social worker, serve as the liaison between the patient and other health care providers and help the patient negotiate these various tasks.

Potential problems in the use of psychotropic agents is an issue both during and following the pregnancy, given the teratogenicity of several psychotropic agents (e.g., lithium) and the fact that some are secreted in high concentrations in breast milk. General recommendations concerning psychotropic drug use in pregnancy are included in the chapter on reproductive health (Chapter 2).

Schizophrenia in mothers is associated with increased rates of fetal and neonatal death (Mednick et al. 1971). Therefore, delivery should be planned for a setting where both intensive psychiatric and obstetrical services are available depending on what complications may develop (Rieder et al. 1975). Elective cesarean section should be considered when the severity of the psychosis makes it likely that the patient will not be able to cooperate adequately in the delivery process. After delivery several additional issues surface, including the capacity of the mother to adequately care for the child, potential problems in bonding between the mother and infant, and the possible need for foster home placement.

Many women with schizophrenia who become pregnant and are not married choose to give up their children for adoption or to place them in foster care. Obviously such plans should be set in motion as early in the pregnancy as possible and appropriate, and, once again, court involvement, often through child protection agencies, may be necessary.

PROBLEMS IN DELIVERING MEDICAL CARE TO PATIENTS WITH SCHIZOPHRENIA

The medical management of patients with schizophrenia can be quite difficult (Bunce et al. 1982). One of the major problems is difficulty in communication between the psychiatric patient and the medical caregivers. This is illustrated by a report from Pary and Barton (1988), who studied a series of 110 psychotic patients, 38 of whom had a total of 54 medical problems listed on Axis III at index hospitalization. The 38 patients were followed up approximately 2 years later; 1 had died and 2 had moved away and were unavailable. Of the remaining 35 patients, 28 agreed to participate. Twenty-four (86%) were unable to name at least one of the physical problems with which they had been diagnosed during the index hospitalization.

Many patients with chronic psychosis, even those with severe illness that may produce intense pain, do not seem to complain of discomfort and at times will ignore such conditions as fractures, third-degree burns, and perforated ulcers (Talbott and Linn 1978). This observation seems to correspond with the literature on pain insensitivity in schizophrenia, which is frequently observed but currently little understood. This phenomenon has recently been reviewed by Dworkin (1994), who concludes that the literature supports the observation that some patients with schizophrenia indeed have alterations in pain perception. Whether this is a central or peripheral nervous system difference is unclear.

Massie (1989) outlined steps in the management of schizophrenic patients with cancer; these recommendations seem applicable to schizophrenic patients with any chronic medical illness:

1. The patient will tend to cooperate best if he or she is managed solely by one physician and one health care team. It is also useful to have a social worker who can act as a liaison among the clinic and hospital staff, the family, and the patient.
2. A psychiatrist should be involved in the patient's care on an ongoing basis and may have to work closely with the nursing staff on management of behavioral problems.

3. Work with the family, if available, is often critical. Family members will have to assume much of the responsibility for care at home, including giving medications and scheduling clinic visits. The alternative is a close liaison with the psychiatric caregivers.
4. Severely disturbed patients should have a single person who is available for visits and telephone contact. Massie (1989) suggested that this person use a supportive psychotherapy approach and provide frequent contact.

SUMMARY

Patients with schizophrenia may experience a variety of medical problems complicating their psychosis and may also present challenges in the management of concurrent medical problems. Physicians should be alert to the known complications of schizophrenia, especially self-injury, foreign-body ingestion, and polydipsia with water intoxication. Furthermore, other diseases may occur with increased or decreased frequency in comparison with the general population, and their management may be more difficult in the patient with schizophrenia. Close contact between the psychiatrist and other medical personnel is critical in providing the optimal management of these patients.

REFERENCES

Adler LE, Griffith JM: Concurrent medical illness in the schizophrenic patient: epidemiology, diagnosis, and management. Schizophr Res 4:91–107, 1991

Akasaki Y, Nagatomo I, Akasaki Y, et al: Water intoxication in a schizophrenic patient with rhabdomyolysis. Japanese Journal of Psychiatry and Neurology 4:843–846, 1993

Alroe CJ, Gunda V: Self-amputation of the ear: three men amputate four ears within five months. Aust N Z J Psychiatry 29:508–512, 1995

Altom RL, DiAngelis AJ: Multiple autoextractions: oral self-mutilation reviewed. Oral Surg Oral Med Oral Pathol 67:271–274, 1989

Babigian HM, Odoroff CL: The mortality experience of a population with psychiatric illness. Am J Psychiatry 126:470–480, 1969

Baldwin JA: Schizophrenia and physical disease (editorial). Psychol Med 9:611–618, 1979

Birrer RB, Robinson T, Rao S, et al: Self-mutilation: three cases and a review of the literature. J Emerg Med 11:27–31, 1993

Blacker KH: Four cases of autocastration. Arch Gen Psychiatry 8:79–86, 1963

Buda M, Tsuang MT, Fleming JA: Causes of death in DSM-III schizophrenics and other psychotics (atypical group): a comparison with the general population. Arch Gen Psychiatry 45:283–285, 1988

Bunce DFM II, Jones LR, Badger LW, et al: Medical illness in psychiatric patients: barriers to diagnosis and treatment. South Med J 75:941–944, 1982

Burgess HA: Schizophrenia in pregnancy. Issues Health Care Women 2:61–69, 1980

Crowder JE, Gross CA, Heiser JF, et al: Self-mutilation of the eye. J Clin Psychiatry 40:420–423, 1979

Culliford L: Autocastration and biblical delusions in schizophrenia. Br J Psychiatry 150:407, 1987

Cutting J: Physical illness and psychosis. Br J Psychiatry 135:109–119, 1980

Daniels SM, Fenley JD, Powers PS, et al: Self-inflicted burns: a ten-year retrospective study. J Burn Care Rehabil 12:144–147, 1991

de Leon J, Verghese C, Tracy JI, et al: Polydipsia and water intoxication in psychiatric patients: a review of the epidemiological literature. Biol Psychiatry 6:408–419, 1994

de Leon J, Dadvand M, Canuso C, et al: Polydipsia and water intoxication in a long-term psychiatric hospital. Biol Psychiatry 1:28–34, 1996

Dworkin RH: Pain insensitivity in schizophrenia: a neglected phenomenon and some implications. Schizophr Bull 20:235–248, 1994

Ehrentheil OF: Common medical disorders rarely found in psychotic patients. Archives of Neurology and Psychiatry 77:178–186, 1957

Emsley R[A], Potgieter A, Taljaard F, et al: Water excretion and plasma vasopressin in psychotic disorders. Am J Psychiatry 146:250–253, 1989

Emsley RA, Spangenberg JJ, Roberts MC, et al: Disordered water homeostasis and cognitive impairment in schizophrenia. Biol Psychiatry 9:630–633, 1993

Emsley R[A], Roberts M, Smith R, et al: Disordered water homeostasis in schizophrenia and cerebral ventricular size. Br J Psychiatry 4:501–506, 1995

Favazza AR: Why patients mutilate themselves. Hosp Community Psychiatry 40:137–145, 1989

Feldman MD: The challenge of self-mutilation: a review. Compr Psychiatry 29:252–269, 1988

Fleischhacker WW, Barnas C, Ledochowski M: Hyponatremia-induced organic mental disorder may mask paranoid schizophrenia. Biol Psychiatry 22:650–652, 1987

Garcia-Estrada A: Self-inflicted eye injuries. Br J Psychiatry 153:266, 1988

Goff DC, Henderson DC, Amico E: Cigarette smoking in schizophrenia: relationship to psychopathology and medical side effects. Am J Psychiatry 149:1189–1194, 1992

Goldman MB, Nash M, Blake L, et al: Do electrolyte-containing beverages improve water imbalance in hyponatremic schizophrenics? J Clin Psychiatry 4:151–153, 1994

Gopalaswamy AK, Morgan R: Smoking in chronic schizophrenia. Br J Psychiatry 149:523, 1986

Hall DC, Lawson BZ, Wilson LG: Command hallucinations and self-amputation of the penis and hand during a first psychotic break. J Clin Psychiatry 42:322–324, 1981

Herpertz S: Self-injurious behaviour: Psychopathological and nosological characteristics in subtypes of self-injurers. Acta Psychiatr Scand 91:57–68, 1995

Hughes JR, Hatsukami DK, Mitchell JE, et al: Prevalence of smoking among psychiatric outpatients. Am J Psychiatry 143:993–997, 1986

Hussar AE: Leading causes of death in institutionalized chronic schizophrenic patients: a study of 1,275 autopsy protocols. J Nerv Ment Dis 142:45–57, 1966

Jacob B, Huckenbeck W, Barz J, et al: Death, after swallowing and aspiration of a high number of foreign bodies, in a schizophrenic woman. Am J Forensic Med Pathol 11:331–335, 1990

Kampmeier RH: Diagnosis and treatment of physical disease in the mentally ill. Ann Intern Med 86:637–645, 1977

Katz J, Kunofsky S, Patton RE, et al: Cancer mortality among patients in New York mental hospitals. Cancer 20:2194–2199, 1967

Kennedy BL, Feldmann TB: Self-inflicted eye injuries: case presentations and a literature review. Hosp Community Psychiatry 45:470–474, 1994

Kikoler DJ, Duberstein DL, Zagoren AJ, et al: A large accumulation of metallic foreign bodies in the stomach. J Am Osteopath Assoc 92:657–660, 1992

Krasucki C, Kemp R, David A: A case study of female genital self-mutilation in schizophrenia. Br J Med Psychol 68:179–186, 1995

Langbehn DR, Pfohl B: Clinical correlates of self-mutilation among psychiatric inpatients. Ann Clin Psychiatry 5:45–51, 1993

Lipper S, Werman DS: Schizophrenia and intercurrent physical illness: a critical review of the literature. Compr Psychiatry 18:11–22, 1977

MacLean G, Robertson BM: Self-enucleation and psychosis. Arch Gen Psychiatry 33:242–249, 1976

Martin T, Gattaz WF: Psychiatric aspects of male genital self-mutilation. Psychopathology 24:170–178, 1991

Massie MJ: Schizophrenia, in Handbook of Psychooncology. Edited by Holland JC, Rowland JH. New York, Oxford University Press, 1989, pp 287–310

Masterson E, O'Shea B: Smoking and malignancy in schizophrenia. Br J Psychiatry 145:429–432, 1984

Mednick SA, Mura E, Schulsinger F, et al: Perinatal conditions and infant development in children with schizophrenic parents. Soc Biol 18:S103–S113, 1971

Muqtadir S, Hamann MW, Molnar G: Management of psychotic pregnant patients in a medical-psychiatric unit. Psychosomatics 27:31–33, 1986

Nakaya M: On background factors of male genital self-mutilation. Psychopathology 29:242–248, 1996

O'Sullivan ST, Reardon CM, McGreal GT, et al: Deliberate ingestion of foreign bodies by institutionalized psychiatric hospital patients and prison inmates. Ireland Journal of Medical Sciences 4:294–296, 1996

Osterberg E: Schizophrenia and rheumatic disease: a study on the concurrence of inflammatory joint diseases and a review of 58 case-records. Acta Psychiatr Scand 58:339–359, 1978

Pary RJ, Barton SN: Communication difficulty of patients with schizophrenia and physical illness. South Med J 81:489–490, 1988

Paterson AJ, Stewart F, Tulloch EN: Self-inflicted mutilation of the dentition in a schizophrenic patient. Br Dent J 173:314–316, 1992

Rieder RO, Rosenthal D, Wender P, et al: The offspring of schizophrenics: fetal and neonatal deaths. Arch Gen Psychiatry 32:200–211, 1975

Shore D, Anderson DJ, Cutler NR: Prediction of self-mutilation in hospitalized schizophrenics. Am J Psychiatry 135:1406–1407, 1978

Shutty MS Jr: Cigarette use, drinking, and voiding in schizophrenic patients with polydipsia and hyponatremia. Schizophr Res 3:195–197, 1996

Slovis CM, Tyler-Werman R, Solightly DP: Massive foreign object ingestion. Ann Emerg Med 11:433–435, 1982

Spielvogel A, Wile J: Treatment of the psychotic pregnant patient. Psychosomatics 27:487–492, 1986

Talbott JA, Linn L. Reactions of schizophrenics to life-threatening disease. Psychiatr Q 50:218–227, 1978

Tobias CR, Turns DM, Lippmann S, et al: Evaluation and management of self-mutilation. South Med J 10:1261–1263, 1988

Vieweg WV: Treatment strategies in the polydipsia-hyponatremia syndrome. J Clin Psychiatry 55:154–160, 1994

Vieweg WV, Pandurangi A, Levenson J, et al: The consulting psychiatrist and the polydipsia-hyponatremia syndrome in schizophrenia. Int J Psychiatry Med 24:275–303, 1994

Vieweg WV, Levenson J, Pandurangi A, et al: Medical disorders in the schizophrenic patient. Int J Psychiatry Med 25:137–172, 1995

Weiser M, Levy A, Neuman M: Ear stuffing: an unusual form of self-mutilation. J Nerv Ment Dis 181:587–588, 1993

Witherspoon CD, Feist FW, Morris RE, et al: Ocular self-mutilation. Ann Ophthal 21:255–259, 1989

Young LD, Feinsilver DL: Male genital self-mutilation: Combined surgical and psychiatry care. Psychosomatics 27:513–517, 1986

5

Munchausen's Syndrome and Other Factitious Disorders

INTRODUCTION

Patients with factitious disorders feign physical symptoms or intentionally produce organic illness, with their sole aim being the assumption of the patient role (Folks 1995; Folks and Freeman 1985; Jones 1995; Morris 1991; Pankratz 1981; Plassman 1994; Plewes and Fagan 1994; Reich and Gottfried 1983; Sutherland and Rodin 1990; Wise and Ford 1999). These patients must be distinguished from malingerers, who simulate illness for the purpose of an obvious secondary gain, such as financial compensation or avoidance of unpleasant duties (Eisendrath 1996). Patients with factitious illness may either fabricate symptoms or signs of illness, for example, by manipulating thermometers to erroneously indicate a febrile response, or may artificially induce actual organic illness, for example, by self-inoculation of contaminated materials into intravenous lines. This latter behavior can obviously result in life-threatening complications. However, all forms of the disease can be dangerous if the unwary clinician orders unnecessary diagnostic or therapeutic procedures, each of which may carry a small but definite iatrogenic risk. Patients with factitious disorders often demand substantial physician attention and use many medical resources before being discovered (Powell and Boast 1993; Schlesinger et al. 1989), placing themselves at risk of medical complications and potentially depriving other patients of needed health care attention.

DEFINITION AND OVERVIEW OF FACTITIOUS DISORDERS

DSM-IV-TR (American Psychiatric Association 2000) classifies factitious disorders into two major categories (Table 5–1): factitious disorder (divided into three subtypes depending on whether there are predominantly physical or psychological signs and symptoms, or both) and factitious disorder not otherwise specified (which includes factitious disorder by proxy).

Table 5–1. DSM-IV-TR criteria for diagnosis of factitious disorders

Factitious disorder
Intentional production or feigning of physical or psychological signs or symptoms
Motivation is to assume sick role
External incentives (such as economic gain, avoiding legal responsibilities, or improving physical well-being, as in malingering) are absent
Three subtypes of factitious disorder
With predominantly psychological signs and symptoms
With predominantly physical signs and symptoms
With combined psychological and physical symptoms
Factitious disorder not otherwise specified
Includes disorders with factitious symptoms that do not meet the criteria for factitious disorder, for example, factitious disorder by proxy: the intentional production or feigning of physical or psychological signs or symptoms in another person who is under the individual's care, for the purpose of indirectly assuming the sick role.

Source. American Psychiatric Association 2000

Munchausen's syndrome refers to a factitious disorder in which physical signs and symptoms predominate. It is usually characterized by dramatic simulation of disease states, pathological lying, and peregrination or wandering (Asher 1951; Spiro 1968). The true incidence of factitious illness is unclear due to difficulties in establishing a diagnosis and the tendency for patients to receive care at multiple institutions (American Psychiatric Association 2000; Folks 1995).

Traditionally, Munchausen's syndrome has been recognized in men of lower socioeconomic status with borderline personality traits and poor social functioning (Carney 1980; Ireland and Sapira 1967); more recent reports have emphasized that women, especially those with a medical background, may present with a factitious disorder (Folks and Freeman 1985; Freyberger et al. 1994; Jones 1995; Plewes and Fagan 1994; Reich and Gottfried 1983). Typically, patients with factitious illness repeatedly seek medical attention (Fink and Jensen 1989), often with dramatic presentations and medically sophisticated stories (Epstein 1995). When the factitious nature of the problem is suspected, patients will often leave the medical facility and move to a new physician or hospital, and the cycle will begin anew (Jones 1995). In the extreme, patients may undergo hundreds of hospitalizations and spend most of their days in the hospital.

MEDICAL COMPLICATIONS

Although the vast majority of patients with factitious illness are cared for by nonpsychiatric physicians when they present with medical complaints, some are appropriately transferred to a psychiatrist for management after the diagnosis of factitious disease has been recognized. It is critical for psychiatrists to remember that these patients will often continue to feign or induce medical illnesses and that such illnesses often require medical intervention. The health care team must work together to correctly differentiate feigned illnesses from self-induced diseases that require medical management and from intercurrent true medical problems. In the case of feigned illness, it is important to avoid ordering extensive diagnostic testing, making unnecessary referrals, or attempting empiric therapeutic interventions. In contrast, self-induced illnesses can result in true organic diseases that require transfer to a medical or surgical physician.

Patients with Munchausen's syndrome often present with multiple manifestations of factitious illness. Although one diagnosis or organ system may be favored, patients may switch "illnesses," complaining of several different types of self-induced disease. Thus, it is imperative that the psychiatrist be familiar with the various medical complications of Munchausen's and other factitious disorders—quite a challenge considering that these patients can be very creative and will undoubtedly continue to invent as-yet-undescribed manifestations of illness.

In the original description of Munchausen's syndrome, three major types of cases were identified: abdominal, hemorrhagic, and neurological (Asher 1951). Since then, many additional manifestations of Munchausen's syndrome, simulating organic illnesses in virtually all organ systems, have been recognized (Freyberger et al. 1994; Nordmeyer 1994; Plassman 1994) (Table 5–2).

Table 5–2. Medical manifestations of factitious disorders

Hematologic

Anemia—self-bloodletting, self-induced trauma, ingestion of drugs
Factitious bleeding—hemoptysis, hematuria, gastrointestinal bleeding
Simulation of sickle cell crises
Self-induced anticoagulation—abuse of warfarin

Infectious diseases

Factitious fever—due to thermometer manipulation, injection of materials to cause infection or inflammation, self-exposure to known allergens
Self-induced infections
False claims of HIV/AIDS

Oncologic

False claims of malignant disease

Cardiologic

Feigned ischemic chest pain
Dysrhythmias—feigned by manipulation of recording devices, self-induced by ingestion of cardiac drugs
Self-induced elevations of blood pressure

Dermatologic

Self-injury to prevent wound healing
Exposure of skin to known irritants, allergens

Endocrinologic

Diabetes—feigned, failure to take insulin in diabetics
Hypoglycemia—abuse of insulin, sulfonylureas; feigned symptoms
Cushing's—abuse of prednisone
Thyrotoxicosis—abuse of thyroid supplements
Hypercalcemia—due to illicit use of vitamin D preparations

Gastrointestinal

Feigned abdominal pain
Bleeding—self-induced trauma, feigned blood loss
Diarrhea—ingestion of laxatives, feigned symptoms
Drug-induced colitis

Pulmonary

Hemoptysis—self-induced trauma, feigned blood loss
False claims of pulmonary embolus symptoms
Laryngeal obstruction, simulation of asthma

Genitourinary

Urinary tract infection—self-inoculation, manipulation of urine culture results
Hematuria—self-induced trauma, manipulation of urine samples
Bartter's syndrome—abuse of diuretics, laxatives, licorice

Table 5–2. Medical manifestations of factitious disorders *(continued)*

Neurologic
Feigned seizures
Feigned paralysis/sensory loss, simulation of cerebrovascular accidents, brain tumors, brainstem dysfunction, multiple sclerosis, subarachnoid hemorrhage
Feigned syncope
Feigned meningitis/encephalitis
Feigned mental retardation
Traumatic
Self-induced multiple trauma due to accidents

Hematologic Manifestations

Hematologic Munchausen's is one of the most common forms of factitious illness (Zahner and Schneider 1994). Patients with Munchausen's syndrome soon learn that medical attention can be quickly garnered in the face of apparent bleeding from the lungs, gastrointestinal tract, or genitourinary system (Chapman 1957). Hemoptysis, hematemesis, colonic bleeding, and hematuria can all be feigned or self-induced. Factitious bleeding is most often accomplished by collecting blood, either by autovenipuncture, exsanguination of animals, or surreptitious procurement of blood products from the hospital, and injecting or ingesting the blood, pouring it on clothes (Feinsilver et al. 1983), or adding it to urine or stool samples (Ifudu et al. 1992). Patients may simulate gastrointestinal bleeding to create a false positive endoscopy or red cell–labeled isotope scan by ingesting the blood (McIntyre and Kamm 1990) or giving themselves blood by enema (Bakkers et al. 1985). Other patients will self-induce blood loss, for example by cutting the tongue or oral cavity to mimic hemoptysis or hematemesis, traumatizing the urethra to induce hematuria, or causing perianal tears to simulate gastrointestinal blood loss with guaiac-positive stools.

Other hematologic forms of Munchausen's are well documented. Probably the most common is self-induced anemia (Daily et al. 1963). This is usually accomplished by autovenipuncture (Granacher 1982), with some patients creating sufficient blood loss to necessitate transfusions. Other patients may ingest drugs, such as arsenic (Abram and Hollender 1974), methotrexate (Ford et al. 1984) or alkylating agents (Ford et al. 1984) that are known to suppress red blood cell production.

One of the best-documented causes of hematologic Munchausen's syndrome is self-medication with oral anticoagulants (Abram and Hollender 1974; Agle et al. 1970; Lazarus and Kozinn 1991; O'Reilly and

Aggeler 1976). These patients frequently are nurses or others with medical training or employment. Patients may have a history of (appropriate) treatment with oral anticoagulant medications. They usually present with laboratory test results suggesting coagulation abnormalities. Although patients may be asymptomatic, extensive and expensive medical evaluations may be ordered. In other cases, serious bleeding complications, including spontaneous hemorrhage, can result (O'Reilly and Aggeler 1976).

Other hematologic illnesses may be feigned by the patient with Munchausen's syndrome. For example, factitious sickle cell anemia with episodes of painful crises has been described (Ballas 1996; Lindenbaum 1974).

Cardiologic Manifestations

A wide variety of cardiac diseases have been simulated by patients with Munchausen's syndrome. Chest pain purported to be angina pectoris is the most common cardiac symptom with which Munchausen's patients present (Cavenar et al. 1980; Dickinson and Evans 1987; Fink and Jensen 1989; Nordmeyer 1994). Patients are most often male and present to emergency rooms complaining of "crushing, substernal chest pain" (Kounis 1979; Pitt and Pitt 1984). Given the difficulty in ruling out myocardial infarction and the potentially dire consequences of a missed diagnosis, most physicians will admit these individuals to the coronary care unit, where the patient willingly assumes the sick role. This can be taken to dramatic extremes—for example, one patient repeatedly flew on commercial airliners and developed "chest pain," necessitating diversion of the airplanes for emergency landings (Addison and Talan 1974). Indeed, invasive diagnostic investigations are often recommended for patients with cardiac Munchausen's syndrome, and these can be associated with adverse consequences. For example, one patient underwent repeated cardiac catheterization, which was eventually complicated by ventricular fibrillation and later by left brachial occlusion resulting in amputation of the left arm below the elbow (Shah et al. 1982).

Another often-reported manifestation of cardiac Munchausen's syndrome is the simulation of cardiac dysrhythmias. Patients may manipulate cardiac monitor electrodes in order to produce rhythm strips that erroneously appear to represent ventricular tachycardia or fibrillation (Ludwigs et al. 1994). In one case, the patient, a physician, would shake the cardiac monitor to mimic tracings consistent with ventricular fibrillation and then deliberately hyperventilate to cause loss of consciousness and apnea (Nordmeyer 1994), thus simulating cardiac arrest. Other reported behavior includes tampering with Holter monitor devices to produce pseudobradycardia (Mitchell and Frank 1982) or other abnormal cardiac rhythms. Patients may feign syncope during these attacks and may even be treated with unnecessary insertion of cardiac pacemakers (Cavenar et al. 1980; Ludwigs et al. 1994).

Finally, patients may abuse medications to induce true cardiac symptoms (Nordmeyer 1994), such as the case of a young woman who presented with recurrent cardiovascular collapse due to surreptitious ingestion of propanolol (Warwick and Boulton-Jones 1989). Another patient with chronic atrial fibrillation/flutter repeatedly visited emergency departments demanding, and often receiving, electrical cardioversions, which would only transiently restore sinus rhythm (Tizes 1977).

Gastrointestinal Manifestations

A variety of gastrointestinal presentations have been reported in patients with factitious illness (Nordmeyer 1994). Patients may claim marked abdominal pain (Epstein 1995; Ireland and Sapira 1967), often fortified by histories of past intra-abdominal pathology such as peptic ulcer disease or recurrent pancreatitis. Munchausen's patients may augment these presentations by tampering with laboratory samples by adding blood to stool samples to mimic gastrointestinal bleeding or contaminating urine samples with saliva to generate apparent hyperamylasuria (Nordmeyer 1994). As mentioned earlier, patients may also artificially place blood in the gastrointestinal tract or induce traumatic bleeding to simulate hematemesis or melena. In one case, a patient injected blood into the abdominal wall during a nuclear medicine study in which red blood cells were tagged, thus producing false evidence of gastrointestinal bleeding (Bakkers et al. 1985). The clinician may respond with orders for diagnostic tests and even initiate treatment pending the results of the evaluation. Some patients undergo repeated laparotomies, resulting in the classic "gridiron" abdomen (Jones 1995).

Other forms of gastrointestinal Munchausen's syndrome have been described. Perhaps the most frequent, and one of the more difficult to recognize, is the use of laxatives to induce diarrhea (Ewe and Karbach 1986). A wide variety of laxatives can be abused, ranging from stool softeners to mineral oil (Kramer and Pope 1964; Rosenblum et al. 1977). Acutely, laxative abuse can cause diarrhea, which may prompt the physician to order invasive endoscopy or other tests. Laxative-induced diarrhea can cause electrolyte disturbances, including dehydration and pseudo–Bartter's syndrome (hypertrophy of the juxtaglomerular cells in the kidney, resulting in hypokalemic alkalosis and dysregulation of fluid status). Prolonged laxative abuse can cause malabsorption with consequent malnutrition. Eventually, laxative abuse can cause chronic gastrointestinal dysfunction, including decreased peristalsis and laxative dependence. Less frequently reported gastrointestinal manifestations of Munchausen's syndrome include instillation of caustic soda to induce inflammatory colitis (Byrne et al. 1975) and ingestion of foreign objects such as razor blades, requiring endoscopic or surgical removal (Fink and Jensen 1989). Patients may simulate symptoms of inflammatory bowel disease and then be erroneously treated, even with parenteral nutrition or surgical intervention (Klein et al. 1995).

Neurologic Manifestations

Myriad neurologic presentations have been described in patients with Munchausen's syndrome (Bauer and Boegner 1996; Eckhardt 1994). Patients may feign seizures to gain medical attention (Bauer and Boegner 1996; Christensen and Szlabowicz 1991; Jones and Horrocks 1987). These "seizures" may be so convincing that patients are placed on anticonvulsants despite normal electroencephalograms (Ries 1980). Paralysis and sensory loss may also be claimed by Munchausen's patients (Bauer and Boegner 1996; Quest and Hyler 1980; Ries 1980; Schlesinger et al. 1989; Will and Miller 1992). One individual with chronic asymmetry of his pupils repeatedly feigned unconsciousness and hemiparesis, recurrently prompting neurosurgical evaluation (Fink and Jensen 1989). Other patients may use mydriatic eye drops to create asymmetric pupils (Board and Hammond 1980). Complaints of headache and limb weakness can prompt the physician to order computerized tomography scans to rule out the possibility of a subarachnoid hemorrhage (Will and Miller 1992). One patient with chronic facial paresis repeatedly presented stating that this was a new symptom, resulting in evaluation for possible acute brainstem dysfunction (Fraim and Peters 1979). Simulated amnesia has been reported (Sussman et al. 1987). False claims of fainting and syncope with loss of consciousness are also common (Bauer and Boegner 1996; Bernstein et al. 1991) and may be accompanied by dramatic, fabricated stories such as losing consciousness while landing an airplane (Folger et al. 1981). Patients with Munchausen's syndrome can even effectively simulate cases of meningitis and encephalitis (Marchant and Brown 1990). In addition, true meningitis can subsequently result from iatrogenic complications of diagnostic procedures such as lumbar punctures or myelograms (Robinson and Latham 1987). A patient who effectively faked mental retardation in an apparent attempt to gain admission to adult foster care has been described (Clemmons et al. 1982).

Infectious Disease Manifestations

Factitious fever is recognized as the most common factitious symptom (Murray 1979; Petersdorf and Bennet 1957; Sarwari and Mackowiak 1997). Numerous ingenious methods have been used by patients to record falsely elevated body temperatures (Rumans and Vosti 1978). Patients may place thermometers near heaters, shake thermometers to record a desired temperature, switch thermometers, or rinse their mouths with hot water immediately prior to oral temperature taking. Factitious fever should be considered if the normal circadian variation in temperature is not observed, if tachycardia and diaphoresis do not accompany the fever, or if fever in adult patients is greater than 105°F. Use of electronic thermometers, direct observation of the patient while taking the temperature, or simultaneous measurement of urine and body temperatures can facilitate discovery of the subterfuge (Aduan et al. 1979). In up to 10% of patients with prolonged unexplained fevers, the diagnosis is actually factitious fever (Petersdorf and Bennett 1957). Unfortunately, the diagnosis is often not considered until after extensive and costly evaluation.

Patients may also inject or ingest pyrogenic materials or microbes to induce organic disease and real fevers (Aduan et al. 1979). The substances with which Munchausen's patients inject themselves are quite remarkable, and include tetanus toxoid, feces, saliva, laboratory cultures of bacteria or fungi, or proteins such as milk (Aduan et al. 1979). Patients may inject the foreign materials intravenously, either directly or via catheter, or subcutaneously. In one case, a laboratory technician inoculated herself with a culture of *Mycobacterium tuberculosis* and then deliberately prolonged her recovery by failing to take antituberculous medications prescribed for her disease (Aduan et al. 1979). Self-inoculation should be suspected particularly in the patient with polymicrobial infections that reflect normal colonic or mouth flora (Lazarus and Kozinn 1991) or when infection recurs despite adequate antibiotic therapy. Recurrent skin or soft-tissue abscesses without apparent medical cause should also prompt consideration of self-inoculation.

Ingestion of drugs known to cause fever may be the cause of factitious fever. Patients may also take antibiotics, diphenylhydantoin, quinidine, or other drugs in the face of known allergies to induce fevers.

Recently, a new form of Munchausen's syndrome has been recognized: patients who falsely claim to be infected with HIV or to have AIDS (Churchill et al. 1994; Cottam et al. 1991; Gockel et al. 1990; Harry and Ong 1995; Miller et al. 1986; Robinson and Latham 1987; Ryan et al. 1995; Zuger and O'Dowd 1992). It has been suggested that in some instances, patients falsely purport to have AIDS in order to access specialized medical and social support services that have been implemented to serve this population (Mileno et al. 2001). It is also quite likely that these individuals have learned that many clinicians will have a lower threshold for ordering diagnostic tests and/or hospitalizing patients who are HIV seropositive. In other reports, patients with HIV infection have been noted to feign symptoms of known AIDS complications, such as gastrointestinal bleeding or Kaposi's sarcoma (Cooke and Grace 1990).

Dermatologic Manifestations

Munchausen's patients may also fake a variety of skin lesions (Ormsby 1915). One patient applied reddish makeup in a malar distribution to simulate the "butterfly" rash characteristic of systemic lupus erythematosis (Ifudu et al. 1992). Recurrent skin abscesses may be induced by self-inoculation with foreign substances, such as feces, saliva, milk proteins, and drugs. A variety of self-inflicted injuries have been described (Sneddon and Sneddon 1975), including skin lesions induced by caustic substances such as lye, phenol, and acids (Ormsby 1915). Patients may actually create ulcers or lacerations (Agris and Simmons 1978); nonhealing wounds may be attributable to intentional retraumatization of the involved tissues (Serafin et al. 1983; Tunbridge 1969). Tragically, some of these patients may require amputation (Thomas 1937). In another scenario, a patient with a known skin allergy to thimerosol was discovered to be repeatedly applying the drug to his skin, eventually requiring repeated hospitalizations for severe exfoliative dermatitis (Chapman 1957).

Pulmonary Manifestations

Multiple case reports attest to the frequency of respiratory presentations of Munchausen's syndrome (Hirshberg and Wuerz 1999; Nordmeyer 1994). Because patients have some voluntary control of their own breathing pattern, many abnormal findings can be simulated. Patients often present with dyspnea, which may be accompanied by tachypnea or even stridor (Patterson et al. 1974). Patients can simulate wheezing by voluntarily opposing the vocal cords and may be erroneously diagnosed with asthma (Baker and Major 1994); they may then receive repeated treatments in emergency departments or hospitals (Downing et al. 1982). Feigned or self-induced pulmonary disease can be so apparently severe that patients receive mechanical ventilation. In one reported case, a young woman was able to induce functional paralysis of the right diaphragm and was repeatedly hospitalized. She eventually had a tracheotomy performed for her feigned respiratory problems (Roethe et al. 1981). Another patient was intubated on several occasions for breathing against a closed glottis (Epstein 1995). A more frequent pulmonary presentation of Munchausen's syndrome is deliberate hyperventilation to induce syncope, tetany, and sometimes loss of consciousness (Nordmeyer 1994). Patients with self-inflicted pneumothoraces as a manifestation of Munchausen's syndrome have been reported (Urschel et al. 2001).

Respiratory symptoms may also be induced by the injection, ingestion, or aspiration of microbes to cause pneumonia and other respiratory tract infections. Less frequently, known allergens may be ingested or inhaled to induce bronchospasm in patients with underlying true asthma. Patients may also manipulate tracheostomy sites to induce bleeding or infection (Pender and Pender 1980; Roethe et al. 1981). One patient dyed her skin blue and feigned unconsciousness, thus convincing her physicians that she was cyanotic, until alcohol skin preparation for an intravenous line removed the dye—and the "cyanosis" (Kellner and Eth 1982).

As reviewed earlier, Munchausen's patients will often feign or self-induce hemoptysis (Baktari et al. 1994). Dramatic presentations of blood on the clothing or bedsheets are relatively frequent manifestations of Munchausen's syndrome (Asher 1951). Patients may acquire their own blood by autovenipuncture or obtain blood samples from other sources to produce the "evidence" of hemoptysis. In other cases, patients may injure their oral mucosa to simulate coughing up of blood, in some cases using razor blades to cut the tongue or intravenous catheters to traumatize the oral mucosa (Baktari et al. 1994; Roethe et al. 1981). Patients may augment the presentation of hemoptysis by simulating the symptoms of a pulmonary embolus (Trew and Anderson 1970), often resulting in diagnostic tests and empiric anticoagulation therapy (Roethe et al. 1981), with all their attendant risks.

Genitourinary Manifestations

Many genitourinary symptoms can be mimicked by patients with factitious disorder (Heimbach and Bruhl 1995). Feigned hematuria is a frequent manifestation of Munchausen's syndrome. Patients may adulterate urine samples with their own blood or with blood obtained from other sources. Alternatively, patients may self-medicate with anticoagulants, cause traumatic lesions, or insert foreign objects or substances into the genitourinary tract with consequent trauma or inflammation to produce true hematuria (Kerr et al. 1980). Other patients may add microbes or protein-containing substances to the urine sample to simulate bacteruria or proteinuria (Nordmeyer 1994). When these measures are accompanied by feigned symptoms, patients can fool the physician into making a diagnosis of urinary tract infection or renal stones (Gluckman and Stoller 1993; Rabin and Graham 1984). The latter often requires elaborate investigation to detect the subterfuge. In one case, Munchausen's was proven only when the patient with supposed recurrent renal stones was given radioactive labeled stones on discharge and later presented with a purportedly newly passed stone found to contain the radioactivity (Atkinson and Earll 1974). Patients with adulterated urine samples may succeed in persuading health care providers to initiate diagnostic workups looking for real pathology (Tojo et al. 1990), including malignant lesions. In one case, a patient eventually convinced her physicians to perform a nephrectomy with removal of a normally functioning kidney (Kerr et al. 1980).

Other renal illnesses may be erroneously diagnosed in Munchausen's syndrome. Case reports of simulated lupus nephritis and Goodpasture's syndrome have appeared, including one in which the patient was treated with oral steroids and gold injections for lupus before the true cause was discovered (Ifudu et al. 1992). By ingesting large amounts of diuretics, laxatives, or licorice, patients may induce a pseudo–Bartter's syndrome, manifested by dehydration, electrolyte abnormalities, hyperaldosteronism, edema formation, and, eventually, renal compromise (Rosenblum et al. 1977).

Reports of gynecological Munchausen's syndrome are less common (Fliegher 1983). In one report, two women complained of irregular vaginal bleeding and then altered serum and urine samples to indicate the presence of beta hCG, simulating malignant trophoblastic disease (Board and Hammond 1980).

Oncologic Manifestations

Munchausen's patients may claim to have cancer (D'Andrea 1978), and they are sometimes successful in accessing enrollment in oncology clinics and procuring surgical interventions and chemotherapeutic treatments (Bruns et al. 1994). Patients have falsely claimed to have acute myelogenous leukemia (Reich and Gottfried 1983), Hodgkin's disease (Pendlebury 1991), ovarian cancer (Bruns et al. 1994), laryngeal cancer (Pender and Pender 1980), Kaposi's sarcoma (Cooke and Grace 1990), and metastatic uterine cancer (Baile et al. 1992). These patients often mobilize significant community support for their illnesses. They can consume significant health care dollars in clinicians' attempts to conclusively establish a diagnosis. Convincing stories of missing pathology reports or lost hospital records are often proffered by patients attempting to get medical attention for falsified claims of malignancy. In some cases, chemotherapy, radiotherapy, or surgical evaluation is initiated before the truth becomes known to the duped oncologist. Needless to say, the potential for untoward side effects from these unnecessary interventions is great and places the patient at significant risk for true, albeit iatrogenic, disease.

Endocrinologic Manifestations

Most endocrine presentations of Munchausen's syndrome are attributed to self-medication with drugs that simulate illnesses. Patients may ingest sulfonylurea drugs (Jordan et al. 1977) or use insulin injections (Jermendy 1996) to cause hypoglycemia (Marks and Teale 1999). Surreptitious use of these agents can result in seriously low blood glucose levels and the attendant consequences of decreased level of consciousness and even death. In some cases, covert use of insulin continues even after the patient is hospitalized, such that patients require continuous glucose infusions (Grunberger et al. 1988). A few patients have even been subjected to partial pancreatectomy in a futile search for an occult insulinoma. Conversely, a case of factitious diabetes has been reported in which the patient "spiked" finger-prick blood samples with glucose solutions and took glucagon prior to clinic visits to simulate diabetes; the patient continued to use insulin despite being informed that she did not have diabetes (Kurtz et al. 1979). Other patients who do have diabetes will intentionally withhold insulin to induce hyperglycemia, requiring repeated hospitalizations for diabetic ketoacidosis (Schade et al. 1985).

Abuse of thyroid hormone supplements has been described as causing thyrotoxicosis (Gorman et al. 1970; Rose et al. 1969). Such abuse can cause sudden death, presumably as a result of cardiac arrythmias or drug-induced myocarditis (Bhasin et al. 1981). Truly hypothyroid patients may present a medical enigma when they fail to take prescribed replacement hormones and remain hypometabolic despite claims that they are compliant with their medication regimens (Gorman et al. 1970). Factitious hypercalcemia can be produced by ingesting calcium tablets or vitamin D preparations (Nordmeyer 1994). Surreptitious self-administration of epinephrine has resulted in "factitious pheochromocytoma" (Keiser 1991), in some cases with adrenalectomy being performed. Factitious Cushing's syndrome has been described and attributed to surreptitious use of glucocorticoids (Villanueva 2000). In one interesting case, an adolescent girl ingested large amounts of oral steroid preparations, resulting in apparent Cushing's disease. She hoped to persuade her physicians to perform an adrenalectomy, which she was sure would reverse her long-standing obesity (Witt and Ginsberg-Fellner 1981). In another case, a woman fabricated an elaborate tale of having been diagnosed with systemic lupus erythematosus and persuaded physicians to provide ongoing prescriptions for oral corticosteroids; she eventually developed a cushingoid appearance and other complications of chronic steroid therapy (Tunbridge 1969).

Surgical/Traumatic Manifestations

Factitious disorders in the field of surgery have been frequently described (de Fontaine et al. 2001; Paar 1994; Papadopoulos and Bell 1999). Patients may present to the trauma unit with superficial injuries and wounds or with overt life-threatening trauma. They may complain of a variety of orthopedic problems in an attempt to coerce the surgeon to perform joint or bone surgery (Dooley et al. 1993). And, of course, the surgeon is often the unwitting recipient of the patient for whom surgery, such as laparotomy or wound repair, is requested.

MECHANISMS BY WHICH PATIENTS INDUCE FACTITIOUS ILLNESS

Patients with factitious illness can produce their symptoms through a variety of different mechanisms (Table 5–3).

Falsification of History on Physical Examination

Patients frequently fabricate medical histories. Not infrequently, purported symptoms reflect those of a true illness the patient had in the past; thus, the patient is attempting to perpetuate his or her role as a patient. Patients with Munchausen's syndrome often are remarkably familiar with the medical manifestations of even relatively obscure illnesses and can create impressive and quite believable stories that prompt the clinician to intervene (Jones 1995; Plewes and Fagan 1994). Patients may give complex and convoluted histories of having obtained prior medical care at a variety of medical facilities. They will report having been diagnosed with serious illnesses by previous physicians and implore the current physician to assume the care of their supposed chronic condition. Patients also may be able to actually produce false physical examination findings. Because many bodily functions are under at least semi-voluntary control,

Table 5–3. Mechanisms by which patients feign or induce factitious illnesses

False histories
- Faked symptoms
- Inaccurate medical histories

False physical examination findings
- Wheezing by voluntary control of vocal cords
- Faked paralysis or loss of sensory function

Falsification of diagnostic evaluations
- Manipulation of cardiac recording devices

Drug ingestion
- Oral anticoagulants, insulin, sulfonylurea agents, thyroid preparations, cardiac drugs, prednisone, alkylating agents, laxatives, diuretics, known allergens

Self-induced trauma
- Self-injection of air, feces, saliva, bacteria, other caustic/toxic substances
- Cuts/abrasions/application of caustic substances to cause skin lesions or bleeding
- Deliberate accidents (motor vehicle accidents, falls, burns)
- Ingestion/insertion of foreign bodies

Failure to treat known medical illnesses
- Asthma, diabetes, connective tissue diseases, others

patients can simulate a wide variety of abnormal findings on physical examination. It is critical that the clinician perform a thorough physical examination to determine if the findings are consistent with true organic illness.

Falsifying or Tampering With Test Results

Patients may alter laboratory test results to suggest the presence of a factitious illness. In addition, patients may submit samples from others with known illnesses and claim that the specimens were in fact obtained from the patient. Patients have transmitted falsified histopathology reports (Bruns et al. 1994), as well as a wide variety of other altered diagnostic evaluation test results. Patients may also falsify the results of diagnostic evaluations.

Drug Exposure

Ingestion, injection, inhalation, or dermal application of drugs and other potentially toxic agents are the major mechanisms by which factitious illness can be induced. The list of drugs that may be abused is quite long. Patients with known allergies or hypersensitivity responses to a variety of agents may deliberately take these agents to induce allergic responses (Egan et al. 1999). When the patient denies use of the drug, the findings may remain unexplained and the physician may be forced to search for evidence of illicit use of medications by screening body fluid samples for evidence of the drug or its metabolites.

Self-Induced Trauma

Patients may be so desperate to attain the sick role that they induce trauma to cause medical illness (Banerjee 1991). Patients may inject themselves with air, feces, saliva, or bacteria to create evidence of illness. Patients will often cut themselves or insert or ingest objects into various body orifices to cause bleeding, infection, obstruction, or inflammation. In some cases, surgical removal of the foreign objects is required to prevent further injury (Howe et al. 1983). In one instance, a patient was found to have injected air under her skin to simulate subcutaneous emphysema (Winans et al. 1983). In this tragic case, the young woman developed proptosis, blindness, exenteration of the right eye, and damage to the left eye before the correct diagnosis was made, after a period of more than ten years. Another woman feigned fever and injected air into soft tissues to simulate "gas gangrene" (Rumans and Vosti 1978). Other patients deliberately involve themselves in motor vehicle accidents, falls, or fires (Hedges et al. 1995), with potentially life-threatening complications when the "accident" escalates out of control.

Failure to Treat Known Medical Illnesses

Another mechanism characteristic of Munchausen's syndrome is seen in patients who have true medical illnesses but then manipulate therapeutic interventions or fail to comply with recommended therapies so that their underlying illness worsens. Failure to take prescribed medications, obtain needed medical monitoring and follow-up, or comply with behavioral changes can all result in deliberate exacerbation of otherwise manageable conditions.

MUNCHAUSEN'S SYNDROME BY PROXY

In the devastating illness of Munchausen's syndrome by proxy, the perpetrator abuses a dependent individual, nearly always a young child, by creating factitious symptoms or laboratory results or by intentionally inducing illness (Donald and Jureidini 1996; Lacey et al. 1993; Meadow 1977; Oyelami et al. 1994; Rosenberg 1987; Schreier and Libow 1993, 1994; Skau and Mouridsen 1995; Wilson 2001). Rarely, adults may be the victims of Munchausen's by proxy, as in the case of one man who tranquilized his wife and girlfriend and then caused the wife's death and later the girlfriend's paralysis by injecting gasoline into their bodies (Sigal et al. 1986). The abuser is most commonly the mother, although cases involving fathers (Makar and Squire 1990), other caregivers (Ben-Chetrit and Melmed 1998), and even health care professionals (Repper 1995) are well substantiated.

Victims can be choked or smothered to induce apnea and sudden infant death syndrome (Meadow 1990; Mitchell et al. 1993; Samuels et al. 1992). Carotid massage has been used to create bradycardia (Porter et al. 1994). Other presentations include poisoning (Meadow 1993; Rogers et al. 1976; Tessa et al. 2001), exsanguination to produce anemia, injection with microbes to induce infectious illnesses, use of laxatives to cause chronic diarrhea (de Ridder and Hoekstra 2000), overdosing with emetics to induce vomiting or diuretics to simulate Bartter's syndrome (Bader 1999; D'Avanzo et al. 1995), inflicting trauma to induce bleeding, application of caustic substances to produce rashes (Schreier and Libow 1994), and provision of drugs to induce seizures (Baldwin 1994; Mullins et al. 1999) or hypoglycemia (Owen et al. 2000).

Tragically, this form of child abuse is characterized by a high incidence of death (Bools et al. 1993; Rosenberg 1987), estimated to be as high as 9% in one major study (Rosenberg 1987). All too often, the true diagnosis is unrecognized. Even if it is recognized, the child is often returned to the care of the abuser. An alarming rate of unexplained illness or death also occurs in the siblings of children thought to be victims of Munchausen's by proxy (Bools et al. 1993; Meadow 1990; Samuels et al. 1992). Nevertheless, with careful monitoring, family reunification may be feasible in some cases (Berg and Jones 1999).

Obviously, there are no direct medical consequences to the person who has the disease of Munchausen's by proxy. It is only the victim who suffers. The victims are not considered to have a psychiatric disease, and therefore a discussion of their medical complications lies outside the purview of this review. However, it is interesting to note that in some cases the child victim accepts the parent's myths regarding the feigned illness and may become an active participant in perpetuating his or her feigned symptoms or parent-induced illnesses (Skau and Mouridsen 1995). Children may subject pets or siblings to the same abusive behaviors to which they were subjected by the parent (Porter et al. 1994). Even if the child survives, adverse long-term outcomes are frequent, with an increased incidence of poor school performance, conduct and emotional disturbances, and frank psychiatric illnesses including depression and anxiety disorders.

An increased incidence of factitious illness in patients with Munchausen's syndrome by proxy (i.e., the perpetrators) has been recognized (Samuels et al. 1992). These patients are also reported to suffer from high rates of eating disorders and self-harming behaviors (Samuels et al. 1992). They are often employed or trained in nursing or other health care–related occupations. Abusers may have a history of multiple psychiatric problems, especially depression, and a history of having been victims of sexual, physical, or emotional abuse themselves.

MEDICAL MANAGEMENT

Accuracy of Psychiatric Diagnosis

Treatment of medical complications in patients with factitious illnesses is made more difficult by the fact that most of these patients repeatedly present to medical facilities without the diagnosis of Munchausen's syndrome being suspected. The average factitious disorder is not accurately diagnosed until 5–10 years after it first manifests (Eisendrath 1994). Because these patients often wander to many hospitals, they can repeatedly present with the same feigned or self-induced symptoms without arousing suspicion about the underlying psychiatric illness. In addition, they often seek care in emergency departments, especially those of teaching institutions, in which they see a different clinician, often an inexperienced trainee, for each visit (Plewes and Fagan 1994). Thus, they are able to perpetuate their inappropriate use of medical resources, often for years.

It is clear that establishing a diagnosis of Munchausen's syndrome is critical to the optimal management of these patients (Freyberger et al. 1994). However, the typical response of the patient, when confronted with evidence of the factitious or self-induced nature of the medical problem, is to deny the accusation and leave the hospital against medical advice. Then, the patient moves on to the next doctor, clinic, or hospital to repeat the process. Thus, health care professionals are often unsuccessful in the area that is most essential to the care of the Munchausen's patient—i.e., identifying the psychiatric pathology and setting limits on the evaluation of and therapy for the patient's complaints.

In patients with suspected factitious illness, other underlying psychiatric diagnoses must be ruled out (American Psychiatric Association 2000). In particular, patients with factitious illness must be distinguished from malingerers. As noted earlier, the patient with factitious illness has as his or her sole motivation the assumption of the patient role. Although the behavior is consciously produced, the motivation reflects a psychiatric conflict and is not conscious (Eisendrath 1994). In contrast, the malingerer fakes symptoms to ensure some secondary gain, such as financial compensation; avoidance of punishment, including jail time; or excuse from responsibilities at home, on the job, or at school.

Factitious disorders must also be distinguished from other illness-affirming behaviors. Conversion reactions, somatization disorders, and hypochondriasis may resemble factitious disorders. However, in these other illnesses, both the production of symptoms and the motivation is unconscious (Eisendrath 1989, 1994). The differential diagnosis may also include depression or an anxiety disorder.

Differentiating Between Feigned and Self-Induced Medical Complications

When patients with Munchausen's present, it is essential to accurately determine the true nature of their complaints. The clinician must differentiate feigned symptoms from true, albeit self-induced, organic illness (Plewes and Fagan 1994). In cases in which symptoms or laboratory abnormalities are faked, the goal should be to identify the symptoms as false and to minimize diagnostic evaluations and empiric therapies. For example, for the patient who fakes hemoptysis with exogenously obtained blood, it is important to not order radiographic procedures to rule out pulmonary embolus. The patient who feigns angina-like chest pain should not undergo invasive cardiac tests. In the classic scenario of the patient who fakes abdominal pain, exploratory laparotomies must be avoided. In contrast, the patient with self-induced illness may require aggressive medical management to avoid morbidity and mortality. Thus, the patient with surreptitious insulin use may have life-threatening hypoglycemia that needs to be aggressively treated. Polymicrobial sepsis secondary to self-inoculation with saliva or feces requires appropriate antibiotic therapy and medical stabilization.

Unfortunately, the distinction between feigned symptoms and self-induced illness can at times be quite difficult. The challenge is complicated by the fact that the same patient who fakes symptoms or adulterates laboratory samples may also present, in some cases even simultaneously, with self-induced organic illness (Plewes and Fagan 1994). The careful clinician must, of course, assume the "worst-case scenario" of organic illness, but must be cognizant of the fact that harm can be done by ordering unnecessary evaluations and treatments.

Detecting Factitious Medical Illness

In some cases, there are approaches that can be recommended for establishing the factitious nature of these patients' presentations (Table 5–4).

First and foremost, the health care worker must be aware of Munchausen's syndrome and be alert to this disorder as a possible diagnosis. A patient's extensive knowledge about the illness or dramatic discussions of past treatment should not prevent the clinician from ensuring the accuracy of the medical diagnosis. Consideration that a patient may be faking symptoms is somewhat contrary to the practice of most health care providers, who assume a relationship of mutual trust with their patients to achieve the goal of relieving pain and suffering. Finally, physicians need to remain cognizant of possible countertransference issues. Patients with factitious illness may attempt to convince the treating physician that he or she is the "only one" smart enough or caring enough to accurately treat their condition. Nevertheless, when patients repeatedly present with undocumentable or apparently self-induced illnesses, it is critical to consider the possibility of factitious illness.

A basic practice that can be used to minimize the chances of being deceived is to insist on documentation of all previous diagnoses as well as results of medical evaluations and past therapies. This is good medical practice for all patients and may be more easily accomplished in the future if electronic records come into wider use. Written records from previous clinicians and hospitals should be obtained when new patients present for care. Ideally, these should not be transported by the patient. Remarkable cases have been reported in which patients have altered their hospital or clinic medical records, including switching names on histopathology reports to falsely record that their biopsy results indicated cancer. It is also useful to personally communicate with previous health care providers to ensure an accurate assessment of past medical care. Such caution will help ensure that the "discovery period" for factitious illness is not repeated by each clinician, allowing health care professionals to avoid repeating unnecessary tests or treatments.

A careful physical examination can also help detect cases of factitious illness. For example, although there are some medical conditions in which fever is not accompanied by tachycardia, factitious fever is especially likely in the patient without concomitant tachycardia and diaphoresis. Factitious fever should also be suspected if temperature readings fail to follow a normal diurnal circadian pattern or if fever is greater than 105°F in an adult (Rumans and Vosti 1978). If factitious fever due to thermometer manipulation is suspected, the temperature should be taken under direct observation. Vital signs should be moni-

Table 5–4. Approaches to distinguish factitious from nonfactitious illnesses

Symptom/Sign/Illness	Method
Recurrent presentations with multiple medical complaints	Assign a primary care medical physician to initially evaluate all patient complaints
	Discourage emergency department visits
	Minimize use of multiple specialist consultants
	Minimize practice of "defensive" medical care, i.e., ordering diagnostic tests/procedures to rule out unlikely illnesses
False histories	Careful review of past records, laboratory reports
	Obtaining records, diagnostic testing results directly from previous physicians, hospitals, and/or outside laboratories
	Direct conversations with previous physicians when possible
False claims of previous diagnoses	
HIV	Confirmatory HIV antibody testing
Sickle cell anemia	Confirmatory hemoglobin electrophoresis
Other	Other confirmatory laboratory/radiologic testing
Feigned symptoms	
Fever (thermometer manipulation)	Direct observation while taking temperature
	Comparing oral, rectal, urine temperatures
	Observing for concomitant tachycardia, diaphoresis during fevers
Wheezing	Formal pulmonary function tests, arterial blood gas testing
False laboratory tests	
Hematuria	Bladder catheterization to obtain fresh urine samples

Table 5–4. Approaches to distinguish factitious from nonfactitious illnesses *(continued)*

Symptom/Sign/Illness	Method
Self-induced illnesses	
Autovenipuncture	Hospital room searches to find needles and other blood-drawing equipment
Self-inoculation with microbes, other foreign materials	Suspect if recurrent polymicrobial bacteremia, especially with oral, fecal flora
	Hospital room searches
Ingestion of diuretics, laxatives, other medications	Blood, urine, stool screens to check for suspected agents, such as diuretics, warfarin, cardiac drugs, sulfonylureas, diphenylhydantoin, etc.
Surreptitious use of insulin (factitious hypoglycemia)	Screening for presence of serum antibodies to porcine or bovine insulin; ratio of insulin to C-peptide levels in peripheral venous blood during hypoglycemia
Surreptitious use of thyroid hormone (factitious thyrotoxicosis)	Radioactive iodine scans (total body)
Self-inflicted injury with manipulation of wounds	Observation
	Casting of arms/hands to prevent behaviors
Self-inflicted injury to cause bleeding	Careful physical examination for evidence of oral lacerations that might simulate hemoptysis, hematemesis; vaginal or urethral injuries that might simulate hematuria or irregular vaginal bleeding; gastrointestinal tract injury that might simulate gastrointestinal bleeding
Munchausen's by proxy	Hospitalization of child
	Camera observation of parent–child interactions in hospital room
	Removal of child from home

tored without warning the patient in advance. In one case, a patient always went to the bathroom immediately prior to having her temperature taken; when she was prevented from doing so, she was unable to heat up her mouth with hot water, and the "fever" disappeared. Finally, taking simultaneous oral and rectal temperatures and testing the temperature of freshly voided urine samples can help detect false temperature elevations (Rumans and Vosti 1978).

Thorough physical examination can detect self-induced lacerations created to falsely suggest hemoptysis, hematuria, hematemesis, or melena (Harrington et al. 1988). On neurological examination, an experienced clinician can detect findings that are inconsistent with supposed anatomical defects. The patient who fakes paralysis but then is able to voluntarily control arm or leg movements to prevent discomfort (i.e., when the arm is dropped it moves safely away from the face) can be identified by a thorough physical examination. If the patient is unexpectedly jolted, he or she may use supposedly paralyzed muscles to keep from falling. Finally, careful examination of skin lesions may reveal needle marks at sites of self-inoculation or even the presence of foreign materials that have been injected.

One controversial mechanism for establishing the diagnosis of faked symptoms or self-induced illness is searches of the hospital room or personal effects (Reich and Gottfried 1983). Such searches can detect needles or sharps used for autovenipuncture or self-injection, medications being taken surreptitiously, or supplies used for manipulating laboratory samples. This information can be critical to establishing a diagnosis of factitious illness. Obviously, however, the imperative to respect the patient's rights, including the right to privacy, must be considered when such actions are being contemplated. Legal consultation is usually appropriate (Reich and Gottfried 1983). Comparable issues are involved in covert surveillance of patients and in the use of "registries" or "blacklists" for use in hospital emergency rooms.

Some medical complications of Munchausen's can be detected by ordering confirmatory laboratory testing. For example, rather than accepting a past diagnosis of HIV infection, many HIV clinics now require testing for HIV antibodies for all new or transferred patients (Zuger and O'Dowd 1992). Analogously, patients who report having sickle cell anemia should have confirmation of the diagnosis by hemoglobin electrophoresis (Ballas 1996). Factitious asthma may be detected with the use of formal pulmonary function tests and arterial blood gas testing (Downing et al. 1982).

In addition, self-induced illness caused by ingestion or injection of unindicated medications can often be detected by testing for the presence of the drug in serum, urine, stool, or other samples. For example, illicit use of diuretics, diphenylhydantoin, and many cardiac drugs can be ascertained by detecting serum drug levels in the patient. Use of porcine or bovine insulin results in the production of anti-insulin antibodies that can be detected in the serum of patients (Kurtz et al. 1979). The ratio of insulin to C-peptide (an indicator of endogenous insulin production) in peripheral venous blood during hypoglycemia can also be used to detect surreptitious exogenous insulin administration and distinguish the cause from insulinoma (Jermendy 1996). Patients with factitious thyrotoxicosis can be evaluated by total-body radioactive iodine scanning; if there is no evidence of endogenous functional thyroid tissue, it is reasonable to conclude that the patient is taking exogenous hormone.

In some instances, the nature of the medical complication can suggest factitious illness. If a patient suffers from repeated bouts of polymicrobial sepsis without an obvious source, it is appropriate to consider the possibility of self-inoculation. The patient with repeated laparotomies in which no intra-abdominal pathology is found may well have factitious illness. The patient with renal colic and apparent hematuria who has repeatedly negative intravenous pyelograms might have feigned symptoms. It is, of course, necessary to distinguish between the patient who has unexplained illness and the one with factitious illness. It may be tempting to justify our lack of knowledge by accusing the patient of "faking." The insightful clinician realizes that there will be instances of illness that are not adequately explained by our current medical knowledge and attempt to distinguish these from factitious complaints.

There is significant controversy about covert surveillance of individuals suspected of having Munchausen's syndrome by proxy (Arterburn 2001). Hidden cameras may detect abuse of children and potentially avert a tragic death (Hall et al. 2000). However, the rights of parents must be considered as well (Beckford-Ball 2000).

Use of Medical Consultation

It is clear that management of medical complications in patients with factitious illness can be a challenge. In the case of feigned symptoms, the psychiatrist and the primary care provider should try to minimize medical interventions. This includes attempting to limit the number of subspecialty consultations that are ordered. However, it is recognized that patients with Munchausen's syndrome are often very convincing and that it may be necessary to obtain expert medical consultation to detect the factitious nature of the illness. Nevertheless, the psychiatrist should try to avoid the practice of "defensive medicine," that is, the ordering of multiple tests and consultations to rule out unlikely diseases. In contrast, aggressive management of self-induced illness may be necessary to avoid morbidity and mortality. It is important to realize that Munchausen's patients may seek physicians inexperienced with the particular feigned illness in an attempt to avoid detection. Therefore, the judicious use of medical consultation may be needed to most appropriately manage the medical complications. Finally, whenever possible, the patient should receive care from only one provider or, alternatively, a limited number of physicians, with the overall care coordinated by one physician, so that behavior patterns can be recognized (Pankratz and Jackson 1994).

Legal Considerations

Patients with factitious illness may interact with the legal system in a number of ways, including filing insurance claims, malpractice suits, or disability applications. This is true even if the patient is not malingering for obvious secondary (financial, legal, or social) gain. The psychiatrist often plays an important role in educating lawyers, judges, and/or juries about factitious disorders (Eisendrath 1996). All physicians should be aware of the distinction between factitious disorders and other conditions such as malingering, conversion, hypochondriasis, or somatization, as well as their potential medical complications, if called on to advise or give testimony in legal cases involving these patients.

PROGNOSIS

Perhaps surprisingly, the risk of death in patients with Munchausen's syndrome is quite low. Only rare fatalities have been reported. Occasionally, death may occur as an untoward effect of the diagnostic workup or therapeutic intervention, or from self-induced illness. Death due to "sudden cardiac death" was reported in a young woman who was presumed to be injecting herself with cornstarch and baker's yeast; an autopsy suggested that death was due to respiratory failure after one of her self-injections (Nichols et al. 1990). Fatalities have also been associated with surreptitious use of insulin with consequent hypoglycemia, and after illicit use of thyroid hormone due to cardiac arrythmias (Bhasin et al. 1981). However, the remarkable fact is the rarity with which these patients do develop fatal complications—perhaps suggesting that they are able to regulate their behaviors to produce symptoms severe enough to prompt medical attention but not to kill them; thus, death would result only after a "miscalculation."

Nevertheless, marked morbidity may occur in patients with factitious illnesses (Sutherland and Rodin 1990). The patient who feigns symptoms or manipulates laboratory samples is obviously not at risk from the behavior itself. However, the feigned medical problems often prompt the ordering of diagnostic tests and empiric treatments that may carry risks. For example, the patient who fakes hematuria may develop an allergic reaction to the dye used for the intravenous pyelogram ordered to rule out nephrolithiasis. The patient who complains of chest pain may undergo needless cardiac catheterization and develop complications of the invasive procedure (Shah et al. 1982). The patient who undergoes multiple laparotomies often develops adhesions and therefore true, organic abdominal pain.

Of even more concern is the patient with self-induced illness. These patients have true organic disease that may cause significant morbidity. Patients with self-induced infections can develop severe polymicrobial sepsis, requiring prolonged antibiotic therapy with the associated risks. Patients who blood-let themselves to cause anemia will develop fatigue and decreased exercise tolerance. Those who precipitate an asthma attack by deliberate exposure to allergens may develop respiratory failure, may have an allergic reaction to the medications used to control their symptoms, or may develop sequelae from chronic use of corticosteroids. Patients with self-inflicted wounds or manipulation of nonhealing wounds may require multiple surgeries and even limb amputation.

Finally, it is important to remember that a diagnosis of Munchausen's syndrome does not preclude the need for medical care. This diagnosis provides no guarantee against true medical problems, be they self-induced, iatrogenic, or true organic diseases unrelated to Munchausen's (Pankratz and Jackson 1994). Tragic cases have been reported in which Munchausen's patients sought medical attention so frequently under false pretenses that none was provided later when it was truly needed (Pankratz and Jackson 1994).

In contrast to these scenarios is the victim of Munchausen's by proxy. Presumably because of the vulnerability of the child or dependent victim, a startlingly high rate of mortality is observed in the victims of Munchausen's by proxy (Meadow 1990). Comparably high death rates are reported in the siblings of the diagnosed child (Samuels et al. 1992). The perpetrator (i.e., the patient with Munchausen's by proxy), by definition, does not suffer from medical complications.

Unfortunately, effective treatments for patients with factitious illnesses are not well defined, and psychiatric intervention is rarely successful in modifying behavior (Sutherland and Rodin 1990; Stern 1980). Confrontation or psychiatric consultation often results in the patient leaving the hospital and seeking care from a new, unsuspecting clinician (Plewes and Fagan 1994; Taylor and Hyler 1993). Patients who are also depressed seem to have a better chance of recovery from Munchausen's (Folks and Freeman 1985), often having a lessening of symptoms when the depression is treated adequately, a finding that underscores the need for a careful assessment for depression and other comorbid symptoms. However, most patients continue their behaviors despite psychiatric intervention. At least in some groups, such as young women—especially those with medical backgrounds and self-inflicted diseases—the behaviors seem to decrease with increasing age. However, the wandering male patient, who is often poorly educated and of lower socioeconomic status and shows evidence of repeated surgeries, is less likely to alter his pattern of seeking medical attention.

SUMMARY

Patients with factitious illness can present with a wide variety of medical complications as manifestations of their underlying psychiatric illness. Patients may feign symptoms, alter laboratory test results, or self-induce illness. Unsuspecting clinicians may unwittingly respond with unnecessary diagnostic evaluations or empiric therapies, and patients with factitious illness may undergo extensive medical and surgical management. Frequently, much money and effort is spent in treating such patients before the true nature of their illness is recognized. When it is and patients are confronted, they will often leave the hospital and repeat the cycle elsewhere. Psychiatrists should be aware of the varied medical manifestations of Munchausen's syndrome, including clues to help detect factitious illness. Diagnostic tests should be limited for the patient with feigned symptoms or manipulated laboratory samples. On the other hand, medical consultation by experienced experts may be necessary to manage the potentially life-threatening complications of self-induced illness. Psychiatrists and other mental health care workers can be of great assistance in managing these patients, both by working directly to modify patient behavior and by working with and helping to coordinate the efforts of other health care practitioners involved in the patients' care.

REFERENCES

Abram HS, Hollender MH: Factitious blood disease. South Med J 67:691–696, 1974

Addison TE, Talan KH: Jet-set Munchausen syndrome (letter). N Engl J Med 291:1195, 1974

Aduan RP, Fauci AS, Dale DC, et al: Factitious fever and self-induced infection: a report of 32 cases and review of the literature. Ann Intern Med 90:230–242, 1979

Agle DP, Ratnoff OD, Spring GK: The anticoagulant malingerer: psychiatric studies of three patients. Ann Intern Med 73:67–72, 1970

Agris J, Simmons CW: Factitious (self-inflicted) skin wounds. Plast Reconstr Surg 62:686–692, 1978

American Psychiatric Association: Diagnostic and Statistical Manual of Mental Disorders, 4th Edition Text Revision. Washington, DC, American Psychiatric Association, 2000

Arterburn T: Using hidden cameras to monitor suspected parental abuse. J Healthc Prot Manage 17:80–87, 2001

Asher R: Munchausen's syndrome. Lancet 1:339–341, 1951

Atkinson RL Jr, Earll JM: Munchausen syndrome with renal stones. JAMA 230:89, 1974

Bader AA, Kerzner B: Ipecac toxicity in "Munchausen syndrome by proxy." Ther Drug Monit 21:259–260, 1999

Baile WF, Kuehm CV, Straker D: Factitious cancer. Psychosomatics 33:100–105, 1992

Baker CE, Major E: Munchausen's syndrome: a case presenting as asthma requiring ventilation. Anaesthesia 49:1050–1051, 1994

Bakkers JTN, Crobach LFSJ, Pauwels EKJ: Factitious gastrointestinal bleeding. J Nucl Med 26:666–667, 1985

Baktari JS, Taskin DP, Small HW: Factitious hemoptysis: adding to the differential diagnosis. Chest 105:943–945, 1994

Baldwin MA: Munchausen syndrome by proxy: neurological manifestations. J Neurosci Nurs 26:18–23, 1994

Ballas SK: Factitious sickle cell acute painful episodes: a secondary type of Munchausen syndrome. Am J Hematol 53:254–258, 1996

Banerjee AK: Trauma and Munchausen's syndrome. Arch Emerg Med 8:217–218, 1991

Bauer M, Boegner F: Neurological syndromes in factitious disorder. J Nerv Ment Dis 184:281–288, 1996

Beckford-Ball J: Patients deserve trust not surveillance cameras. Br J Nurs 9:608, 2000

Ben-Chetrit E, Melmed RN: Recurrent hypoglycaemia in multiple myeloma: a case of Munchausen syndrome by proxy in an elderly patient. J Intern Med 244:175–178, 1998

Berg B, Jones DP: Outcome of psychiatric intervention in factitious illness by proxy (Munchausen's syndrome by proxy). Arch Dis Child 81:465–472, 1999

Bernstein JA, Dykewicz MS, Histand P, et al: Potentially fatal asthma and syncope: a new variant of Munchausen's syndrome in sports medicine. Chest 99:763–765, 1991

Bhasin S, Wallace W, Lawrence JB: Sudden death associated with thyroid hormone abuse. Am J Med 71:887–890, 1981

Board JA, Hammond CB: Factitious trophoblastic disease: Munchausen's mole. South Med J 73:831–832, 1980

Bools CN, Neale BA, Meadow SR: Follow-up of victims of fabricated illness (Munchausen syndrome by proxy). Arch Dis Child 69:625–630, 1993

Bruns AD, Fishkin PA, Johnson EA, et al: Munchausen's syndrome and cancer. J Surg Oncol 56:136–138, 1994

Byrne JS, Carney MWP, Harry DS, et al: Self-induced colitis. Postgrad Med 51:246–249, 1975

Carney MWP: Artefactual illness to attract medical attention. Br J Psychiatry 136:542–547, 1980

Cavenar JO, Maltbie AA, Hillard JR, et al: Cardiac presentation of Munchausen's syndrome. Psychosomatics 21:946–948, 1980

Chapman J: Peregrinating problem patients: Munchausen's syndrome. JAMA 165:927–933, 1957

Christensen RC, Szlabowicz JW: Factitious status epilepticus as a particular form of Munchausen's syndrome. Neurology 41:2009–2010, 1991

Churchill DR, DeCock KM, Miller RF: Feigned HIV infection/AIDS: malingering and Munchausen's syndrome. Genitourin Med 70:314–316, 1994

Clemmons RL, Kenny JT, Lentz GA: Munchausen's syndrome presenting as mental retardation. Md State Med J 21:41–42, 1982

Cooke MW, Grace RH: The modern Munchausen syndrome. J R Soc Med 83:272–273, 1990

Cottam S, Cuthbert C, Parapia L: Munchausen AIDS and hemophilia. Eur J Hematol 46:125, 1991

Daily WJR, Coles JM, Creger WP: Factitious anemia. Ann Intern Med 58:533–538, 1963

D'Andrea VJ: Cancer pathomimicry: a report of three cases. Clinical Psychiatry 39:233–240, 1978

D'Avanzo M, Santinelli R, Tolone C: Concealed administration of frusemide simulating Bartter's syndrome in a 4.5-year-old boy. Pediatr Nephrol 9:749–750, 1995

de Fontaine S, Van Geertruyden J, Preud'homme X, et al: Munchausen syndrome. Ann Plast Surg 46:153–158, 2001

de Ridder L, Hoekstra JH: Manifestations of Munchausen syndrome by proxy in pediatric gastroenterology. J Pediatr Gastroenterol 31:208–211, 2000

Dickinson EJ, Evans TR: Cardiac Munchausen's syndrome. J R Soc Med 80:630–633, 1987

Donald T, Jureidini J: Munchausen syndrome by proxy: child abuse in the medical system. Arch Pediatr Adolesc Med 150:753–758, 1996

Dooley DP, Hodges SD, Kelly JW: Factitious infections in orthopedic patients. Orthopedics 16:816–820, 1993

Downing ET, Braman SS, Fox JM, et al: Factitious asthma: physiological approach to diagnosis. JAMA 248:2878–2881, 1982

Eckhardt A: Factitious disorders in the field of neurology and psychiatry. Psychother Psychosom 62:56–62, 1994

Egan AJ, Tazelaar HD, Myers JL, et al: Munchausen syndrome presenting as pulmonary talcosis. Arch Pathol Lab Med 123:736–738, 1999

Eisendrath SJ: Factitious physical disorders: treatment without confrontation. Psychosomatics 30:383–387, 1989

Eisendrath SJ: Factitious physical disorders. West J Med 160:177–179, 1994

Eisendrath SJ: When Munchausen becomes malingering: factitious disorders that penetrate the legal system. Bull Am Acad Psychiatry Law 24:471–481, 1996

Epstein MS: Munchausen syndrome: case reports and literature overview. Md Med 44:39–43, 1995

Ewe K, Karbach U: Factitious diarrhea. Clin Gastroenterol 15:723–740, 1986

Feinsilver SJ, Raffin TA, Kornei MC, et al: Factitious hemoptysis: the case of the red towel. Arch Intern Med 143:567–568, 1983

Fink P, Jensen J: Clinical characteristics of the Munchausen syndrome. Psychother Psychosom 52:164–171, 1989

Fliegher JR: Munchausen's syndrome and self-induced illness in gynecology. Med J Aust 2:666–667, 1983

Folger WN, Lipton RB, Rovner R: Neurologic Munchausen syndrome. Neurology 31:638–639, 1981

Folks DG: Munchausen's syndrome and other factitious disorders. Neurol Clin 13:267–281,1995

Folks DG, Freeman AM: Munchausen's syndrome and other factitious illness. Psychiatr Clin North Am 8:263–278, 1985

Ford CV, Stein R, Kelly MP, et al: Factitial aplastic anemia. J Nerv Ment Dis 172:369–372, 1984

Fraim CJ, Peters BH: Munchausen syndrome (letter). Ann Neurol 6:138, 1979

Freyberger H, Nordmeyer JP, Freyberger HJ, et al: Patients suffering from factitious disorders in the clinico-psychosomatic consultation liaison service: psychodynamic processes, psychotherapeutic initial care and clinicointerdisciplinary cooperation. Psychother Psychosom 62:108–122, 1994

Gluckman GR, Stoller M: Munchausen's syndrome: manifestation as renal colic. Urology 42:347–350, 1993

Gockel K, Vogelman B, Handy W, et al: Factitious AIDS: a case presentation and review of the literature. Wisconsin Med J 89:633–634, 1990

Gorman CA, Wahner HW, Tauxe WN: Metabolic malingerers: patients who deliberately induce or perpetuate a hypermetabolic or hypometabolic state. Am J Med 48:708–714, 1970

Granacher RP: Autovenipuncture as a cause of factitial anemia. J Nerv Ment Dis 170:308–310, 1982

Grunberger G, Weiner JL, Silverman R, et al: Factitious hypoglycemia due to surreptitious administration of insulin. Ann Intern Med 108:252–257, 1988

Hall DE, Eubanks L, Meyyazhagan LS, et al: Evaluation of covert video surveillance in the diagnosis of munchausen syndrome by proxy: lessons from 41 cases. Pediatrics 105:1305–1312, 2000

Harrington TM, Folks DG, Ford CV: Holiday factitial disorder: management of factitious gastrointestinal bleeding. Psychosomatics 29:438–441, 1988

Harry TC, Ong E: Munchausen's syndrome (HIV infection): a trap for the unwary. Br J Clin Pract 49:271–272, 1995

Hedges BE, Dimsdale JE, Hoyt DB: Munchausen syndrome presenting as recurrent multiple trauma. Psychosomatics 36:60–63, 1995

Heimbach D, Bruhl P: Munchausen's syndrome in urology. Int Urol Nephrol 27:539–545, 1995

Hirshberg AJ, Wuerz RC: Two cases of Munchausen's syndrome presenting as acute respiratory distress. J Emerg Med 17:973–976, 1999

Howe GL, Jordan HW, Lockert EW, et al: Munchausen's syndrome or chronic factitious illness: a review and case presentation. J Natl Med Assoc 75:175–181, 1983

Ifudu O, Kolasinski SL, Friedman EA: Brief report: kidney-related Munchausen's syndrome. N Engl J Med 327:388–389, 1992

Ireland P, Sapira JD: Munchausen's syndrome: review and report of an additional case. Am J Med 43:579–592, 1967

Jermendy G: Hypoglycemia factitia: Munchausen syndrome in diabetes mellitus. J Diabetes Complications 10:223–225, 1996

Jones JR, Horrocks FA: Fictitious epilepsy associated with amnesia. Br J Psychiatry 150:257–258, 1987

Jones RM: Factitious disorders, in Comprehensive Textbook of Psychiatry. Edited by Kaplan HI, Sadack BJ. Baltimore, MD, Williams & Wilkins, 1995, pp 1271–1279

Jordan RM, Kammer H, Riddle MR: Sulfonylurea-induced factitious hypoglycemia: a growing problem. Arch Intern Med 137:390–393, 1977

Keiser HR: Surreptitious self-administration of epinephrine resulting in "pheochromocytoma." JAMA 266:1553–1555, 1991

Kellner CH, Eth S: Code blue: factitious cyanosis. J Nerv Ment Dis 170:371–372, 1982

Kerr DNS, Wilkinson R, Horler AR, et al: Factitious hematuria and urinary tract infection. Arch Intern Med 140:631–633, 1980

Klein J, du Vall GA, Klein S: Pseudo-Crohn's disease with bloody diarrhea: a case of Munchausen's syndrome. Dig Dis Sci 40:226–228, 1995

Kounis NG: Munchausen's syndrome with cardiac symptoms: cardiopathia fantastica. Br J Clin Pract 33:67–72, 1979

Kramer P, Pope CE: Factitious diarrhea induced by phenolphthalein. Arch Intern Med 114:634–636, 1964

Kurtz AB, Harrington MG, Matthews JA: Factitious diabetes and antibody mediated resistance to beef insulin. Diabetologia 16:65–67, 1979

Lacey SR, Cooper C, Runyan DK: Munchausen syndrome by proxy: patterns of presentation to pediatric surgeons. J Pediatr Surg 28:827–832, 1993

Lazarus A, Kozinn WP: Munchausen's syndrome with hematuria and sepsis: an unusual case. Int J Psychiatry Med 21:113–116, 1991

Lindenbaum J: Hemoglobin Munchausen. JAMA 228:498, 1974

Ludwigs U, Ruiz H, Isaksson H, et al: Factitious disorder presenting with acute cardiovascular symptoms. J Intern Med 236:685–690, 1994
Makar AF, Squire PJ: Munchausen syndrome by proxy: father as a perpetrator. Pediatrics 85:370–373, 1990
Marchant B, Brown J: Munchausen meningitis. J R Soc Med 83:532–533, 1990
Marks V, Teale JD: Hypoglycemia: factitious and felonious. Endocrinol Metab Clin North Am 28:579–601, 1999
McIntyre AS, Kamm MA: A case of factitious colonic bleeding. J R Soc Med 83:465–466, 1990
Meadow R: Munchausen syndrome by proxy: the hinterland of child abuse. Lancet 2:343–345, 1977
Meadow R: Suffocation, recurrent apnea, and sudden infant death syndrome. J Pediatr 117:351–357, 1990
Meadow R: Non-accidental salt poisoning. Arch Dis Child 68:448–452, 1993
Mileno MD, Barnowski C, Fiore T, et al: Factitious HIV syndrome in young women. AIDS Read 11:278–282, 2001
Miller F, Weiden P, Sacks M, et al: Two cases of factitious acquired immune deficiency syndrome. Am J Psychiatry 143:1483, 1986
Mitchell CC, Frank MJ: Pseudobradycardia during Holter monitoring: the electronic Munchausen syndrome? JAMA 248:469–470, 1982
Mitchell I, Brummitt J, DeForest J, et al: Apnea and factitious illness (Munchausen syndrome) by proxy. Pediatrics 92:810–814, 1993
Morris M: Munchausen's syndrome and factitious illness. Curr Opin Psychiatry 4:225–230, 1991
Mullins ME, Cristofani CB, Warden CR, et al: Amitriptyline-associated seizures in a toddler with Munchausen-by-proxy. Pediatr Emerg Care 15:202–205, 1999
Murray HW: Factitious fever updated. Arch Intern Med 139:739–740, 1979
Nichols GR, Davis GJ, Corey TS: In the shadow of the Baron: sudden death due to Munchausen syndrome. Am J Emerg Med 8:216–219, 1990
Nordmeyer JP: An internist's view of patients with factitious disorders and factitious clinical symptomatology. Psychother Psychosom 62:30–40, 1994
O'Reilly RA, Aggeler PM: Covert anticoagulant ingestion: study of 25 patients and review of world literature. Medicine 55:389–399, 1976
Ormsby OS: Factitious dermatoses. JAMA 65:1622–1628, 1915
Owen L, Ellis M, Shield J: Deliberate sulphonylurea poisoning mimicking hyperinsulinaemia of infancy. Arch Dis Child 82:392–393, 2000
Oyelami OA, Alhaj AM, Airede IK: Munchausen's syndrome by proxy: a case report and review of literature. Cent Afr J Med 40:222–226, 1994
Paar GH: Factitious disorders in the field of surgery. Psychother Psychosom 62:41–47, 1994
Pankratz L: A review of the Munchausen syndrome. Clin Psychol Rev 1:65–78, 1981
Pankratz L, Jackson J: Habitually wandering patients. N Engl J Med 331:1752–1755, 1994
Papadopoulos MC, Bell BA: Factitious neurosurgical emergencies: report of five cases. Br J Neurosurg 13:591–593, 1999

Patterson R, Schatz M, Horton M: Munchausen's stridor: non-organic laryngeal obstruction. Clin Allergy Immunol 4:307–310, 1974

Pender DJ, Pender UB: Otolaryngologica prevarica: Munchausen's syndrome update and report of a case. Laryngoscope 90:657–660, 1980

Pendlebury SC: Malignant Munchausen's. Med J Aust 155:849–850, 1991

Petersdorf RG, Bennet IL: Factitious fever. Ann Intern Med 46:1039–1062, 1957

Pitt E, Pitt B: Cardiopathica fantastica. Am Heart J 108:137–141, 1984

Plassman R: Munchausen's syndrome and factitious diseases. Psychother Psychosom 62:7–26, 1994

Plewes JM, Fagan JG: Factitious disorders and malingering, in The American Psychiatric Press Textbook of Psychiatry, 2nd Edition. Edited by Hales R, Yudofsky S, Talbott J. Washington, DC, American Psychiatric Press, 1994, pp 623–632

Porter GE, Heitsch GM, Miller MD: Munchausen by proxy; unusual manifestations and disturbing sequelae. Child Abuse Negl 18:789–794, 1994

Powell R, Boast N: The million dollar man: resource implications for the chronic Munchausen syndrome. Br J Psychiatry 253–256, 1993

Quest DO, Hyler SE: Neurosurgical Munchausen's syndrome: case report. Neurosurgery 7:412–414, 1980

Rabin PL, Graham BS: Counterfeit calculi. South Med J 77:304–307, 1984

Reich P, Gottfried LA: Factitious disorders in a teaching hospital. Ann Intern Med 99:240–247, 1983

Repper J: Munchausen syndrome by proxy in health care workers. J Adv Nurs 21:299–304, 1995

Ries RK: DSM-III differential diagnosis of Munchausen's syndrome. J Nerv Ment Dis 168:629–632, 1980

Robinson EN, Latham RH: A factitious case of acquired immunodeficiency syndrome. Sex Transm Dis 14:54–57, 1987

Roethe RA, Fuller PB, Byrd RB, et al: Munchausen syndrome with pulmonary manifestations. Chest 79:487–488, 1981

Rogers D, Tripp J, Bertovim A: Non-accidental child poisoning: an extended syndrome of child abuse. Br Med J 1:793–796, 1976

Rose E, Sanders TP, Webb WL Jr, et al: Occult factitious thyrotoxicosis. Ann Intern Med 71:309–315, 1969

Rosenberg D: Web of deceit: a literature review of Munchausen syndrome by proxy. Child Abuse Negl 11:547–563, 1987

Rosenblum MG, Simpson DP, Evenson M: Factitious Bartter's syndrome. Arch Intern Med 137:1244–1245, 1977

Rumans LW, Vosti KL: Factitious and fraudulent fever. Am J Med 65:745–755, 1978

Ryan J, Taylor CB, Bryant GDR, et al: HIV malingering in the accident and emergency department. J Accid Emerg Med 12:59–61, 1995

Samuels MP, McClaughlin W, Jacobson RR: Fourteen cases of imposed upper airway obstruction. Arch Dis Child 67:162–170, 1992

Sarwari AR, Mackowiak MH: Factitious fever: a modern update. Curr Clin Top Infect Dis 17:88–94, 1997

Schade DS, Drumm DA, Eaton RP, et al: Factitious brittle diabetes mellitus. Am J Med 78:777–784, 1985

Schlesinger RD, Daniel DG, Rabin P, et al: Factitious disorder with physical manifestations: pitfalls of diagnosis and management. South Med J 82:210–214, 1989

Schreier HA, Libow JA: Munchausen syndrome by proxy: diagnosis and prevalence. Am J Orthopsychiatry 63:318–321, 1993

Schreier HA, Libow JA: Munchausen by proxy syndrome: a modern pediatric challenge. J Pediatr 125:S110–S115, 1994

Serafin D, Diamond M, France R: Factitious vesicocutaneous fistula: an enigma in diagnosis and treatment. Plast Reconstr Surg 72:81–87, 1983

Shah KA, Forman MD, Friedman HS: Munchausen's syndrome and cardiac catheterization: a case of a pernicious interaction. JAMA 248:3008–3010, 1982

Sigal LA, Altmark D, Carmel I: Munchausen syndrome by adult proxy: a perpetrator abusing two adults. J Nerv Ment Dis 174:696–698, 1986

Skau K, Mouridsen SE: Munchausen syndrome by proxy: a review. Acta Paediatr 84:977–982, 1995

Sneddon I, Sneddon J: Self-inflicted injury: a follow-up study of 43 patients. Br Med J 3:527–530, 1975

Spiro HR: Chronic factitious illness: Munchausen's syndrome. Arch Gen Psychiatry 18:569–579, 1968

Stern TA: Munchausen's syndrome revisited. Psychosomatics 21:329–336, 1980

Sussman N, Borod JC, Cancelmo JA, et al: Munchausen's syndrome: a reconceptualization of the disorder. J Nerv Ment Dis 175:692–695, 1987

Sutherland AJ, Rodin GM: Factitious disorders in a general hospital setting: clinical features and a review of the literature. Psychsomatics 31:392–399, 1990

Taylor S, Hyler SE: Update on factitious disorders. Int J Psychiatry Med 23:81–94, 1993

Tessa C, Mascalchi M, Matteucci L, et al: Permanent brain damage following acute clonidine poisoning in Munchausen by proxy. Neuropediatrics 32:90–92, 2001

Thomas EWP: Dermatitis artefacta: a note on an unusual case. Br Med J 1:804–806, 1937

Tizes R: The professional cardioversion patient: a new medical and psychiatric entity. Chest 71:434–435, 1977

Tojo A, Nanba S, Kimura K, et al: Factitious proteinuria in a young girl. Clin Nephrol 33:299–302, 1990

Trew P, Anderson DE: Munchausen's syndrome masquerading as pulmonary embolism. Med J Aust 2:637–641, 1970

Tunbridge WMG: Munchausen syndrome. N Engl J Med 280:1130–1131, 1969

Urschel JD, Miller JD, Bennett WF: Self-inflicted pneumothoraces. Ann Thorac Surg 72:280–281, 2001

Villanueva RB, Brett E, Gabrilove JL: A cluster of cases of factitious Cushing's syndrome. Endocr Pract 6:143–147, 2000

Warwick GL, Boulton-Jones JM: Recurrent cardiovascular collapse due to surreptitious ingestion of propranolol. Br Med J 298:294–295, 1989

Will RG, Miller JD: A neurosurgical Munchausen revisited. J Neurol Neurosurg Psychiatry 55:737, 1992

Wilson RG: Fabricated or induced illness in children: Munchausen by proxy comes of age. BMJ 323:296–297, 2001

Winans JM, House LR, Robinson HR: Self-induced orbital emphysema as a presenting sign of Munchausen's syndrome. Laryngoscope 93:1209–1211, 1983

Wise MG, Ford CV: Factitious disorders. Prim Care 26:315–326, 1999

Witt ME, Ginsberg-Fellner F: Prednisone-induced Munchausen syndrome. Am J Dis Child 135:852–853, 1981

Zahner J, Schneider W: Munchausen syndrome in hematology. Ann Hematol 68:303–306, 1994

Zuger A, O'Dowd MA: The Baron has AIDS: a case of factitious human immunodeficiency virus infection and review. Clin Infect Dis 14:211–216, 1992

6

Self-Injurious Behavior

INTRODUCTION

Self-injurious behavior, which is associated with myriad terms (including auto-aggression, focal suicide, self-mutilation, and deliberate self-harm syndrome), is a very complex phenomenon. It may involve a wide range of behaviors, and may be seen in patients from many diagnostic groups. For purposes of simplicity, in this chapter we use the term *self-injurious behavior,* although some have attempted to demarcate *self-mutilation* as a phenomenon occurring primarily in individuals who have nonorganic problems and who are not developmentally disabled, while reserving *self-injurious behavior* for those with organic illnesses and/or developmental disability. A useful definition of self-injurious behavior has been offered by Feldman (1988), and it appears quite adequate for our purposes here: "An individual's intentionally damaging a part of his or her own body, apparently without a conscious attempt to die."

In keeping with the focus of this text, forms of self-injurious behavior commonly encountered in childhood rather than adulthood will not be discussed. This includes such phenomena as battered child syndrome and tantrum attacks (Putnum and Stein 1985), as well as several uncommon but serious disorders that usually are first manifest in childhood or adolescence, including Lesch-Nyhan syndrome, Tourette's syndrome, and childhood autism.

CLASSIFICATION

Different authors have devised various classification schemes for self-injury. For example, Feldman (1988) defines self-injurious behavior as something occurring most commonly among psychotic individuals and those who are mentally retarded rather than a typical behavior engaged in by patients with personality disorders, including borderline personality disorder. Walsh and Rosen (1988) suggest a system of classifying self-mutilation by severity. Type I includes mild forms of the behavior, many of which are socially and culturally acceptable, such as ear piercing. The behaviors progress in severity to Type IV, which would include such extreme phenomena as autocastration and self-enucleation, most commonly seen among patients with psychotic illnesses. Instead of following either of these systems, we approach the problem descriptively, paying particular attention to differences in self-injury among different diagnostic groups.

Pattison and Kahan (1983) described the "deliberate self-harm syndrome." They reviewed 56 published cases of self-injury in detail and offered interesting composite information about these patients. Patients ranged in age from 6 to 75 years with a mean of 23 years, and 78% were under age 30. The mean age of onset for the problem was 17 years. The number of episodes of self-injury varied dramatically, from 1 to more than 100, but in only 27% of the cases were the episodes single, and 66% of the subjects engaged in more than one form of self-injury. Forty-nine percent were male and 51% female. Thirty-six percent had comorbid problems with drug or alcohol abuse. Of importance diagnostically, 41% of the patients were psychotic.

In this series and in other reports, particularly severe forms such as ocular self-injury (including self-enucleation) and genital self-injury (including autocastration) clearly appear to be associated with psychotic illnesses, particularly schizophrenia (Tobias et al. 1988). This literature is dealt with extensively in the chapter on medical complications of schizophrenia (see Chapter 4), and is not reviewed here. Self-mutilation and self-injury outside the context of psychosis are more likely to involve less dramatic and usually less damaging behaviors, with the most common forms being self-cutting (72%), burning (35%), interfering with wound healing (22%), scratching (22%), and hair pulling (10%) (Favazza 1992); however, 8% involve the breaking of bones.

As summarized by Feldman (1988), the arms are the most common site of injury, although any body part can be injured. Although the presence of single or multiple slashes or cuts is the most common pattern, sometimes an individual will carve symbols, names, or initials into the skin (Feldman 1988).

CAUSE AND PREVALENCE

Feldman (1988) cited at least 10 underlying cultural and pathophysiological factors associated with self-injury phenomena, including the following (some paraphrased):

- Ritual symbolism in religion (e.g., culturally bound forms of self-mutilation; these are not addressed here)
- Custom and convention (e.g., ear piercing)
- Psychosis (discussed in Chapter 4)
- Psychodynamic formulsion (center on dynamic formulations of self-mutilation as an attenuated form of suicide)
- Secondary gain (e.g., attention seeking)
- Contagion and conformity (e.g., the "clustering" of self-injury in a center for disturbed adolescents as documented by Walsh and Rosen [1985])
- Adaptation (e.g., a prisoner wishing to change his environment)
- Regression (e.g., head banging, body rocking, and other rhythmic patterns, particularly in those with developmental disabilities)
- Rage
- Organic causes (e.g., Lesch-Nyhan and other biological abnormalities, including those mentioned earlier in this chapter). This category also includes self-injury occurring in the context of drug intoxication, a classic example being face picking and laceration in individuals abusing amphetamines.

The prevalence of self-injury is far from clear. Citing various literature, Walsh and Rosen 1988 postulated an overall incidence range from 14 to 600 per 100,000 individuals per year, while Tantam and Whittaker (1992) offered a figure of 1 in 600 adults.

FORMS OF PSYCHOPATHOLOGY AND SELF-INJURY

Self-injury clusters in those with Axis II personality disorders, particularly borderline personality disorder, and at times among individuals with antisocial features, particularly those who are incarcerated. Self-injury also occurs in certain developmentally disabled populations, particularly among those with relatively severe retardation. The association with borderline personality disorder has frequently been noted in descriptive accounts of this condition; considerable research was concentrated on this relationship in the 1970s (Gunderson and Kolb 1978; Gunderson and Singer 1975). Schaffer et al. (1982) compared 14 self-mutilating patients with 14 psychiatric control subjects and found much higher rates of borderline personality disorder (10 vs. 2) in the self-mutilators. Simeon et al. (1992) compared 26 self-mutilating individuals with personality disorder with 26 nonmutilating control subjects with personality disorder.

Those who engaged in self-mutilation had more character pathology and scored higher on measures of regression and antisocial behavior.

The second clinical condition that is commonly associated with self-injurious behavior is developmental disability. Singh (1981), in a review of the literature, indicated that the prevalence of self-injurious behavior in institutionalized mentally retarded individuals was 5.3%–37.1%, but changes in demographics and rates of institutionalization since then have probably affected the incidence. Given the higher severity of disability in patients who remain institutionalized today, it is possible that the rates are now higher.

Walsh and Rosen (1985) also reviewed the issue of self-mutilation and pointed out that this behavior is much more likely to be frequent and repetitive in self-mutilating individuals with mental retardation than in those without mental retardation. They also point out that tools such as knives and scissors are rarely used by the developmentally disabled, and that these individuals instead engage in head banging, biting, scratching, slapping, or punching. There is some suggestion that such problems may be particularly prevalent in the profoundly retarded (Russ 1992).

The third condition frequently associated with self-injury is antisocial personality disorder. This is particularly so among patients who are incarcerated (Virkkunen 1976). The prevalence of these behaviors in such individuals has not been established, but self-injury does seem to correlate with other psychological problems and behaviors, such as drug and alcohol abuse, rage attacks, fighting, and social withdrawal. Foreign-body ingestion as a means of self-injury, often involving an attempt to manipulate staff, has also been reported in this population (O'Sullivan et al. 1996).

OTHER FACTORS

Descriptively, the definition of self-injury usually includes the proviso that it must result in observable tissue damage. However, self-injury has a low lethality and should not be confused with suicide attempts. It is usually performed in isolation and is often associated with feelings of anxiety, depression, anger, emptiness, and/or alienation (Russ 1992). The behavior itself is frequently motivated by a desire to release tension, and often occurs in those with problems in affect regulation (Herpertz 1995). The role of impulsivity in this phenomenon is less clear. Although self-mutilation can be engaged in impulsively, at other times it is carefully and meticulously planned (Russ 1992).

The pain that results from self-injury is of particular interest in that some patients report no pain at all, whereas others report pain but indicate that the sense of pain is one reason that they engage in the behavior, because it makes them feel "real" or "alive" or allows them to concentrate on something other than their emotional problems. With cutting, much of the focus seems to be on observing flowing blood rather than clotted blood or blood from other sources (e.g., menstrual flow) (Feldman 1988).

MANAGEMENT OF SELF-INJURY

Poisoning/Ingestion

Toxic ingestions are quite common forms of suicidal behavior and are not commonly used by those who chronically injure themselves through self-mutilating behavior. However, the methods used by these two groups of patients can certainly overlap, and a word or two about toxic ingestions would be prudent (Sullivan 1993). An extremely valuable resource is the Regional Poison Center. The National Association of Poison Centers does an excellent job of staffing its phone lines and will answer questions regarding possible ingestions 24 hours a day. In areas not served by a local poison center, calls will be transferred to a regional center that may be some distance away but will be able to help the clinician in a timely fashion.

Acetaminophen ingestion causes the greatest concern from the standpoint of legal liability and missed diagnosis (Sullivan 1993). Acetaminophen is unusual in its ability to be ingested in potentially fatal amounts with minimal clinical symptomatology. Most other medications, when ingested in dangerous amounts, cause at least some symptoms, such as altered level of consciousness, nausea, vomiting, or abnormal vital signs. Most emergency physicians screen all possible overdose patients for acetaminophen. The most valuable screening results are those from tests done 4–6 hours after ingestion. Based on these levels, potential toxicity can be extrapolated and appropriate treatment administered. If the clinician suspects that the patient may have taken an overdose, the situation should be discussed with the poison center or the patient should be referred directly to the emergency department for an evaluation.

One of the most valuable sources of information in these situations is the patients' friends and family. Clinicians should request that friends, family, ambulance personnel, and police search the patient's room or workplace for clues about the ingestion. Looking through garbage cans and wastebaskets, medicine chests, and bedroom drawers will often turn up empty bottles. A good history, including a thorough search of the surroundings, is often much more valuable than serum drug screens. One important reminder about acetaminophen and aspirin is that these two words are commonly thought by patients to be synonymous. It is common for a physician to get a report of a patient overdosing on "aspirin" only to find that it was actually acetaminophen, and vice versa. Therefore, routine screening for both drugs is appropriate.

There are several strategies for treating the patient with a suspected overdose. Ipecac has been almost completely abandoned by most toxicologists due to its marginal efficacy. However, it still may be useful in a few situations, primarily when the ingested substance cannot be absorbed by charcoal. For example, lithium is not absorbed by charcoal and is appropriately treated by ipecac-induced emesis, especially if this can be accomplished in the first hour after ingestion. Most other ingestions should be treated with charcoal. One recent addition to the armamentarium is charcoal based in a sorbitol solution, which prevents constipation and contains a flavoring agent of cherry syrup.

Blunt Trauma

Blunt trauma is certainly less common than lacerations as a type of self-injury, but occasionally does occur. When there is suspicion that the damage may be significant (marked bruising, any significant distortion of the anatomy, suggestion of fracture), arrangements should be made for evaluation in an emergency department. The main factor in determining the level of diagnostic intervention necessary in head trauma is neurologic status (Valadka and Narayan 1996). Evaluation of neurologic status immediately after the injury and also at the time of the examination is extremely helpful in guiding the need for computed tomography (CT) scanning. Skull X rays are rarely beneficial unless there is a question of a foreign body or a depressed skull fracture, and CT scanning is the modality of choice. If a patient has no neurologic symptoms, no alteration in level of consciousness, and no significant headache either at the time of the accident or at the time of the examination, no imaging is needed. If there are abnormal neurologic findings at any time after the injury or at the time of the examination, a CT scan is indicated.

Neck injuries can be difficult to evaluate (Thal 1996). The safest option is referral to the emergency department, especially if the patient is having any significant neck pain or neurologic symptoms. If the patient is alert and awake, has no distracting injury (such as a broken extremity elsewhere), is not intoxicated, and does not have midline tenderness on palpation of the spinous processes of the cervical spine, diagnostic imaging is not needed. Patients with neck stiffness but no midline tenderness may have a whiplash type of injury. Unlike tenderness in the paraspinal or the sternocleidomastoid muscles, any tenderness in the midline should prompt radiographic imaging of the cervical spine. If the patient is uncooperative, is intoxicated, or has an altered level of consciousness, diagnostic imaging should be undertaken if the history prompts any concern regarding spinal injury. With this protocol, unnecessary cervical spine X rays can be avoided. A normal set of cervical spine X rays does not rule out unstable spinal injury. The patient with significant neck pain and/or any neurologic symptoms who has a normal cervical spine X-ray series should still undergo CT scanning.

Torso trauma is primarily found in falls from a height and in motor vehicle accidents (Mattox et al. 1996). Self-injury with trauma to the torso is certainly uncommon but can occur. Generally if the patient has any respiratory difficulty or any significant tenderness of the abdomen following trauma, diagnostic imaging is advisable.

With regard to extremity trauma, the need for radiographic evaluation is determined primarily by symptoms. If a patient has suffered an injury to an arm, leg, hand, or foot, the need for emergency department evaluation can be determined primarily by the patient's functional ability. For example, with lower-extremity trauma, if a patient can ambulate without significant pain, it is unlikely that X rays are necessary. For any distal sensory or circulatory abnormality in an extremity, urgent evaluation is recommended.

Lacerations

The most common site of self-inflicted laceration tends to be the volar surface of the forearm near the wrist (Simon and Brenner 1994). Typically, these wounds are transverse, although some patients will choose the more potentially dangerous longitudinal approach. Even with very deep wounds, exsanguination is unlikely to result from transverse lacerations. If the ulnar or radial artery is severed completely, the vessel will usually spasm and clot after a short period of time. Most deep wounds in this area can be stabilized with direct pressure.

A common question among psychiatric providers is which wounds can be safely managed in the office and which need referral.

If a patient has had multiple previous lacerations in the region and has a significant amount of scar tissue, management of the wound is dictated primarily by function, with a focus on prevention of infection and less concern about cosmetic effects. Tape-strip closure can be considered if two requirements are met. It is necessary to ensure first that the wound is adequately cleansed and second that the edges can be reasonably approximated with the tape strips. Initial management consists of gentle wound cleansing using 4×4 gauze and a non-ionic detergent. Once the wound is cleansed, it can be assessed to see whether the wound edges can be closed. Wound closure tape strips are best used with a skin glue such as Mastisol. Tincture of benzoin has been most commonly used over the years and is commonly available. However, Mastisol does have some advantages over tincture of benzoin; Mastisol is much less likely to cause an allergic reaction, and its ability to secure tape strips is better than that of benzoin. Mastisol is applied to intact skin a few millimeters from the wound and allowed to dry. Tape strips are applied by initially securing them to half of the wound and then gently pulling the tissue closed and placing the strips on the other half of the wound. If the wound seems to be adequately closed in this fashion, it can be dressed with a padded dressing such as 4×4 bandages and gauze wrap. If the wound edges do not come together in a reasonable fashion, suturing is advisable. One of the problems with tape strip closure is that the wound edges tend to roll and become inverted rather than everted. The fastest and strongest wound healing takes place when the wound edges are everted, so that the epithelial surfaces do not fold in against each other. If a wound can be closed with tape strips without a lot of wound edge inversion, it should heal properly. If, however, the edges persistently roll inward, the wound will heal poorly and more aggressive wound management may be needed.

One caveat regarding wound management is that of time. If psychiatric intervention is desirable for a patient with a self-inflicted injury, the definitive closure of most extremity wounds can be delayed. Of course, getting an initial cleansing done is a good idea, but at that point the wound can be protected with a gauze bandage if psychiatric intervention is desirable. Certainly, the earlier the wound is managed definitively, the better.

Most important, with any extremity wound, is checking distal neurologic and circulatory function. Checking to see if a patient has complete sensation in and use of all muscle groups distal to the injury is important to document, as is adequate circulation. If there has been a large amount of bleeding, an arterial injury should be suspected. If the patient with a pulsatile bleeding extremity presents in the office, the bleeding can generally be controlled with direct pressure. If this is not successful, a blood pressure cuff can be placed proximal to the wound and inflated up to the patient's systolic blood pressure to form a tourniquet. This is much safer and gentler on the tissues than is the old-style band type of tourniquet, which is not advisable.

One concern with all open wounds is tetanus status. In a situation in which the patient is being evaluated in psychiatric offices, general guidelines for a tetanus booster should be available. It should be noted, however, that this is not an emergent issue and can safely be taken care of within 24–48 hours. If a patient has not had a tetanus immunization within 10 years, a booster is advisable. If a wound is grossly contaminated and the patient's tetanus immunization is out of date, then a combination of tetanus immune globulin and tetanus toxoid booster is advisable. With some dirty wounds, one can administer tetanus toxoid, if the time since the last booster has been over 5 years. A current trend in emergency medicine is the strong consideration of more liberal use of tetanus immune globulin when wounds have significant devitalized tissue. In this situation, however, most wounds of this type will end up being referred to the emergency department.

The bottom line on treatment of volar forearm lacerations by psychiatric staff could be summarized as follows: Good cleansing is advisable. Office staff can be prepared to handle this type of injury by making sure that there is a ready supply of examination gloves available for staff protection. A couple of boxes of 4×4 gauze dressings serve the dual purpose of allowing for wound cleansing as well as for dressing in a temporizing fashion. If the wound is of significant depth or if there is any hint of distal sensory, motor, or circulatory dysfunction, the patient should be referred to the emergency department. If wounds are superficial and can be brought together with tape strip closure, they can certainly be managed in an office setting.

An additional note about wound-cleansing substances concerns more powerful cleansers such as Hibiclens and Betadine. Both of these products can be used to clean intact skin but should not be used in an open wound. Both are tissue toxic and result in more tissue inflammation than desired. Therefore, if these products are in your office, they are useful for cleaning the hands of staff prior to taking care of a wound and fine for cleaning the skin around a wound, but they should not be used inside a wound. The non-ionic detergent Shur-Clens is preferable in that it is an excellent cleanser but is completely tissue neutral and safe to use inside wounds.

If a practice includes a large number of patients who engage in self-injurious behaviors, the staff may consider having a physician's assistant or another member of the staff spend some time in a local emergency department. Here, staff can obtain the training necessary to more aggressively manage at least minor wounds in the office. However, one must be cautious with regard to wound management around the hand and wrist. If there is any question as to possible tendon, nerve, or artery involvement, then the patient should be referred to an emergency department.

SUMMARY

Self-injurious behavior is a very complex phenomenon. Causes range from symbolic, ritualistic self-mutilation, to self-injury in the context of psychosis, to self-injury in the service of secondary gain. In terms of comorbid psychopathology self-injury clusters among those with Axis II personality disorders, particularly borderline personality disorder, and in a subgroup of those individuals with developmental disabilities.

The management of self-injury depends on the nature of the injury. Toxic ingestions are common forms of suicidal behavior, but can also be used among those who are attempting to injure themselves. Trauma is less common than lacerations, but is a type of self-injury that occasionally does occur. The most common site of self-inflicted laceration tends to be the volar surface of the forearm, near the wrist. Suggestions for the medical management of this type of injury are reviewed.

REFERENCES

Favazza AR: Repetitive self-mutilation. Psychiatr Ann 22:60–63, 1992

Feldman MD: The challenge of self-mutilation: a review. Compr Psychiatry 29:252–269, 1988

Gunderson JG, Kolb JE: Discriminating features of borderline patients. Am J Psychiatry 135:792–796, 1978

Gunderson JG, Singer MT: Defining borderline patients: an overview. Am J Psychiatry 132:1–13, 1975

Herpertz S: Self-injurious behaviour: psychopathological and nosological characteristics in subtypes of self-injurers. Acta Psychiatr Scand 91:57–68, 1995

Mattox KL, Wall MJ Jr, Pickard LR: Thoracic trauma: general considerations and indications for thoracotomy, in Trauma, 3rd Edition. Edited by Feliciano DV, Moore EE, Mattox KL. Stamford, CT, Appleton and Lange, 1996, pp 345–353

O'Sullivan ST, Reardon CM, McGreal GT, et al: Deliberate ingestion of foreign bodies by institutionalized psychiatric hospital patients and prison inmates. Irish Journal of Medical Sciences 165:294–296, 1996

Pattison EM, Kahan J: The deliberate self-harm syndrome. Am J Psychiatry 140:867–872, 1983

Putnam N, Stein M: Self-inflicted injuries in childhood. Clin Pediatr 24:514– 517, 1985

Russ MJ: Self-injurious behavior in patients with borderline personality disorder: biological perspectives. J Personal Disord 6:64–81, 1992

Schaffer CB, Carol J, Abramowitz SI: Self-mutilation and the borderline personality. J Nerv Ment Dis 170:468-480, 1982

Simeon D, Stanley B, Frances MD: Self-mutilation in personality disorders: psychological and biological correlates. Am J Psychiatry 149:221–226, 1992

Simon RR, Brenner BE: Emergency Procedures and Techniques. Baltimore, MD, Williams & Wilkins, 1994

Singh NN: Current trends in the treatment of self-injurious behavior. Adv Pediatr 28:377–382, 1981

Sullivan JB Jr: Poisoning, drug overdose, and toxic exposures, in Emergency Medicine, 3rd Edition. Edited by Kravis TC, Warner CG, Jacobs JLM Jr. New York, Raven, 1993, pp 469–499

Tantam D, Whittaker J: Personality disorder and self-wounding. Am J Psychiatry 161:451–464, 1992

Thal ER: Injury to the neck, in Trauma, 3rd Edition. Edited by Feliciano DV, Moore EE, Mattox KL. Stamford, CT, Appleton and Lange, 1996, pp 329–343

Tobias CR, Turns DM, Lippmann S, et al: Evaluation and management of self-mutilation. South Med J 81:1261–1263, 1988

Valadka AB, Narayan RK: Injury to the cranium, in Trauma, 3rd Edition. Edited by Feliciano DV, Moore EE, Mattox KL. Stamford, CT, Appleton and Lange, 1996, pp 267–278

Virkkunen M: Self-mutilation in antisocial personality (disorder). Acta Psychiatr Scand 54:347–352, 1976

Walsh BW, Rosen PM: Self-mutilation and contagion: an empirical test. Am J Psychiatry 142:119–120, 1985

Walsh BW, Rosen PM: Self-Mutilation: Theory, Research and Treatment. New York, Guilford, 1988

7

Eating Disorders

INTRODUCTION

The eating disorders anorexia nervosa, bulimia nervosa, and binge eating disorder may be associated with serious medical complications (Agras 2001; Becker et al. 1999; Comerci 1990; deZwaan and Mitchell 1992; Mehler 1996a, 1996b; Mitchell et al. 1987a; Palla and Litt 1988; Pomeroy and Mitchell 1989; Sharp and Freeman 1993). These medical complications may involve virtually every major organ system. Careful medical management of these complications is critical to the successful treatment of eating disorders and may be life saving.

Anorexia nervosa is the eating disorder associated with the highest morbidity and mortality (Brown and Mehler 2000; Crisp et al. 1992; Neumarker 1997; Patton 1988; Ratnasuriya et al. 1991). Deaths are most often the result of inanition, suicide, or cardiac events. Early studies suggested mortality rates ranging from 6% to 20%, but more recent studies are conflicting. A few studies suggest that patients who receive treatment may have very low death rates (Strober 1997), but most suggest significant risk of death from causes related to anorexia nervosa (Emborg 1999; Fichter and Quadflieg 1999; Herzog et al. 1997; Zipfel et al. 2000). In one study, the standardized mortality ratio for patients with anorexia nervosa was 6, compared with the general population (Emborg 1999). About 50% of patients recover, 30% improve but have persistent weight-related issues, and 20% have poor outcomes (Becker et al. 1999; Brown and Mehler 2000). Criteria for the diagnosis of anorexia nervosa include failure to maintain body weight greater than 85% of ideal, intense fear of gaining weight, distorted body image, and, in females, amenorrhea.

Bulimia nervosa is less commonly associated with medical complications, but the associated purging behaviors of diuretic, laxative, and ipecac abuse may result in serious illnesses. Criteria for the diagnosis of bulimia nervosa include repeated episodes of consumption of large numbers of calories, feelings of lack of control during binges, and purging behaviors at least twice a week for 2 months. The most recently described eating disorder is binge eating disorder. The medical complications of this disorder, which are less well studied, are predominantly manifested as complications of obesity. Binge eating disorder is defined as recurrent episodes of binge eating behavior without purging.

SYMPTOMS AND SIGNS OF EATING DISORDERS

Most patients with eating disorders will not present to health care providers complaining of symptoms attributable to the eating disorder and in fact may attempt to conceal evidence of the disorder from the health care provider. The history of caloric restriction or bingeing and purging will often not be revealed. If the patient is presenting for evaluation because other family members are concerned about the possibility of an eating disorder, the patient may be particularly resistant to discussion.

In anorexia nervosa, the symptoms and signs are usually those that occur secondary to caloric restriction and weight loss (Table 7–1).

Although anorectic patients will rarely complain about disordered eating, they may be concerned about other symptoms such as cold intolerance, abdominal pain, or abnormal hair growth. On physical examination, evidence of excessive weight loss is usually the most prominent finding. Unfortunately, because of society's emphasis on thinness, both family members and physicians may fail to recognize the seriousness of the patient's condition. Health care workers should not be fooled by attempts to conceal weight loss, such as wearing baggy clothes or artificially inflating weight with hidden objects. Most of the physical manifestations of anorexia nervosa are similar to the abnormalities observed in patients with starvation due to other causes. However, there are a few important differences. For example, most starving patients will note lethargy and inability to exercise, whereas many patients with anorexia nervosa may exercise excessively in attempts to lose weight. Patients with weight loss from other causes will express concern about the weight loss, whereas those with anorexia will minimize, deny, or take pride in their low body weight. Finally, many anorectic patients will deny feelings of hunger, an unusual finding in other forms of starvation.

In contrast to patients with anorexia nervosa, those with bulimia nervosa or binge eating disorder often appear physically healthy (Table 7–1).

Table 7–1. Major symptoms and signs in eating disorders

	Anorexia nervosa	Bulimia nervosa	Binge eating disorder
Symptoms	Denial of illness Amenorrhea Agitation (hyperactivity) Irritability, withdrawal Sleep disturbances, lethargy Fatigue, headaches Constipation Cold intolerance	Secrecy surrounding binge–purge behaviors Irregular menses Abdominal pain Lethargy Constipation Swelling of hands and/or feet Depression	Request for diet advice Eating binges Weight concerns Depression Symptoms due to complications of obesity
Signs	Inanition Low body temperature Bradycardia, hypotension Dry skin, brittle hair, brittle nails Yellow skin, especially palms Lanugo hair Hair loss on scalp Edema	Often appear well Russell's sign Parotid gland swelling Erosion of dental enamel Edema	Often overweight Otherwise usually appear well Signs due to complications of obesity

Bulimic patients may have few symptoms and signs of illness; when present they are usually attributable to purging or associated behaviors of diet pill, diuretic, or laxative abuse. A percentage of these patients are overweight and may present for advice on dieting. Such patients should be carefully interviewed about eating habits (Bruce and Wilfley 1996). Because binge eating is often done secretively, most patients will not provide this information unless specifically asked. In addition, the associated behaviors of purging and laxative, diet pill, diuretic, or ipecac abuse are often concealed from the health care worker. Most often such patients present for medical care with nonspecific complaints, such as bloating, heartburn, constipation, or swelling of the hands and feet. The diagnosis can be easily overlooked if the physician misses these subtle clues.

INITIAL MEDICAL EVALUATION

After an eating disorder is diagnosed, referral to a medical physician familiar with eating disorders for a complete medical history and physical examination is recommended. Some eating disorder programs include a medical physician (usually a family practitioner, internist, pediatrician, or psychiatrist) familiar with the physical manifestations of eating disorders as a member of the treatment team. Although the psychological aspects of the eating disorder may dominate the presentation, it is critical that assessment of the patient's physical status be incorporated into the treatment program. At the initial medical visit, the health care provider should complete a careful medical history and physical examination in a nonjudgmental and caring atmosphere (Table 7–2).

The medical history should include questions that allow the health care provider to assess the severity and chronicity of the eating disorder. Inquiries about dietary habits and weight history should be routine. A review of actual body weights from childhood to the present is critical. Because menstrual irregularities are an important clue to the presence of an eating disorder in women and because prolonged amenorrhea is associated with a high risk of osteoporosis, a careful history regarding menstrual function is important. Given the frequency of comorbid psychiatric conditions, especially depression and chemical dependency, a psychiatric, alcohol, and illicit drug use history is essential. Finally, a particular effort should be made to elicit any history of diuretic, diet pill, or laxative use.

A physical examination should be performed for every patient with a possible eating disorder. The history will provide clues to areas that should be emphasized in the physical examination. Special attention

Table 7–2. Initial medical evaluation of patients with eating disorders

History, with special emphasis on
Weight history
Diet history
Menstrual history (women)/sexual history
Psychiatric history
Chemical abuse/dependency history
Use of diuretics/laxatives/diet pills/ipecac
Physical examination, with special emphasis on
Weight, degree of inanition
State of hydration
Dental examination
Cardiac, abdominal, and neurologic examinations
Gynecologic examination (women)

should be paid to obtaining an accurate height and weight and assessing the degree of inanition or overweight. The state of hydration should be assessed by examination of mucus membranes, skin turgor, and orthostatic blood pressure measurements. In bulimic patients, a careful dental examination to detect dental caries and enamel erosion is paramount. Thorough cardiac, lung, and abdominal examinations may reveal important evidence of medical complications in these organ systems. A screening neurologic examination, including routine screening of visual fields, is important to rule out central nervous system lesions that might mimic eating disorders (Pomeroy and Mitchell 1989). A gynecologic examination is appropriate for all women, with attention paid to detecting possible signs of estrogen deficiency.

Choice of laboratory tests at the initial medical evaluation will be guided by the results of the history and physical examination. Most patients with eating disorders should undergo screening laboratory tests. A complete blood count with differential and determination of serum, electrolytes, blood urea nitrogen, creatinine, glucose, calcium, and liver enzymes are indicated for most patients. Albumin or transferrin may be measured as an indicator of nutritional status. Because the symptoms and signs of both hyper- and hypothyroidism can mimic eating disorders, thyroid function tests are appropriate. Urinalysis and stool guaiac examination are also important. An electrocardiogram with rhythm strip is desirable for some patients, especially severely emaciated anorectic patients and those who have abused diuretics or ipecac. Specific complaints or abnormalities on physical examination may prompt further tests, such as chest or abdominal roentgenograms, electromyography, head computed tomography or magnetic resonance imaging scans, or gastrointestinal endoscopy. In anorectic patients, especially those with prolonged amenorrhea, bone densitometry to assess extent of osteoporosis may be useful. Finally, if diuretic or laxative abuse is suspected but denied by the patient, urine or peripheral blood samples to detect the surreptitious use of these agents can be ordered (Turner et al. 2000).

DIFFERENTIAL DIAGNOSIS OF EATING DISORDERS

Because eating disorders can be mimicked by many other medical conditions, a critical goal of the initial medical evaluation is to rule out other causes of disordered eating. Many of the symptoms and signs of eating disorders can be caused by various underlying medical conditions, and misdiagnosis can result in tragedy. Other illnesses can result in weight loss and mimic manifestations of anorexia nervosa. A careful history and physical examination should detect many of these, especially occult malignancies, chronic infections, diabetes, or malabsorption syndromes. Selected laboratory tests can facilitate diagnosis of other illnesses, such as thyrotoxicosis or renal abnormalities, which may simulate anorexia nervosa.

Similarly, a variety of other medical conditions may present with symptoms that are difficult to distinguish from bulimia nervosa. For example, illnesses such as inflammatory bowel disease and connective tissue syndromes may cause abnormal gastrointestinal motility and mimic many of the symptoms of bulimia nervosa. A careful history to elicit description of self-induced vomiting can prevent protracted, expensive, and uncomfortable evaluations.

Binge eating disorder must be differentiated from genetic or acquired central nervous system abnormalities that result in comparable disordered eating behaviors. However, most of these entities are quite rare, and they are often accompanied by other evidence of pathology. Generally speaking, these diagnoses can be made with a thorough medical history and physical examination and basic laboratory screening tests. Complex and expensive workups are rarely indicated.

MEDICAL COMPLICATIONS

Eating disorders can cause serious, at times fatal, medical complications that can involve all of the major organ systems (Table 7–3).

Table 7–3. Medical complications of eating disorders (by major organ system)

Complication	Related to calorie restriction/ starvation	Related to bingeing/ purging	Related to associated behaviors
Cardiovascular			
Orthostasis/hypotension	X	X	X
Bradycardia	X		
Congestive heart failure	X		X
Electrocardiographic abnormalities	X	X	X
Refeeding cardiomyopathy	X		
Refeeding edema	X		
Arrythmias			X
Sudden cardiac death	X	X	X
Ipecac myocarditis			X
Renal/Electrolytes			
Dehydration; volume depletion	X	X	X
Decreased glomerular filtration rate	X	X	X
Abnormal electrolytes	X	X	X
Kaliopenic nephropathy			X
Refeeding edema	X		
Reflex edema (after stopping laxatives, diuretics)			X
Endocrine			
Growth retardation	X		
Delayed onset of puberty	X		
Abnormal HPG axis, irregular menses, amenorrhea, estrogen deficiency	X	X	
Abnormal HPA axis, sustained hypercortisolism	X		
Abnormal thyroid function tests	X		
Gastrointestinal			
Salivary/parotid gland hypertrophy		X	
Hyperamylasemia		X	
Esophageal perforation/ esophagitis		X	
Mallory-Weiss tears		X	
Delayed gastric emptying	X	X	X
Superior mesentery artery syndrome	X		
Gastric dilatation/rupture		X	

Table 7–3. Medical complications of eating disorders (by major organ system) *(continued)*

Complication	Related to calorie restriction/ starvation	Related to bingeing/ purging	Related to associated behaviors
Refeeding pancreatitis	X		
Constipation	X	X	X
Melanosis coli			X
Steatorrhea/protein-losing gastroenteropathy			X
Cathartic colon			X
Hypokalemic ileus	X	X	X
Metabolic			
Osteoporosis/osteopenia	X		
Trace mineral deficiencies (e.g., zinc)	X	X	X
Vitamin deficiencies (unusual)	X	X	X
Hypercholesterolemia	X		
Obesity (see also Table 7–4)		X	X
Pulmonary			
Subcutaneous emphysema		X	
Pneumomediastinum		X	
Aspiration pneumonitis		X	X
Dermatologic			
Hair loss	X		
Lanugo-like hair growth	X		
Dry skin, brittle hair, nails	X		
Petechiae, purpura (secondary to thrombocytopenia)	X		
Russell's sign (finger calluses and abrasions)		X	
Hematologic/Immunologic			
Anemia	X		
Leukopenia with relative lymphocytosis	X		
Thrombocytopenia	X		
?-Impaired cell-mediated immunity	X		
Abnormal $CD4^{+}/CD8^{+}$ counts	X		
Abnormal cytokines	X		

Table 7–3. Medical complications of eating disorders (by major organ system) *(continued)*

Complication	Related to calorie restriction/ starvation	Related to bingeing/ purging	Related to associated behaviors
Neurologic			
Enlarged ventricles	X		
?—Abnormal pituitary gland size	X		
?—Abnormal electroencephalogram	X	X	
?—Sleep disorders	X	X	
Abnormal positron emission tomography scans	X	X	
Other			
Dental complications		X	
Impaired thermoregulation	X		
Vitamin K deficient coagulopathy	X		
Skeletal muscle myopathy			X

Note. HPA = hypothalamic-pituitary-adrenal; HPG = hypothalamic-pituitary-gonadal.

Cardiovascular

Cardiac abnormalities are frequent in patients with eating disorders (Cooke and Chambers 1995; Dresser et al. 1992; Isner et al. 1985; Kreipe and Harris 1992; Schocken et al. 1989). Case reports indicate that cardiac complications are most likely to occur in very-low-weight anorectic patients and bulimic patients with electrolyte abnormalities resulting from purging or abuse of diuretics or laxatives. In patients with anorexia nervosa, starvation may be associated with sinus bradycardia, sinus arrhythmia, or low blood pressure. These abnormalities are generally considered to be a physiologic adaptation to the hypometabolic state of starvation and are usually not life threatening. Both anorexia nervosa and bulimia nervosa may be associated with dehydration, orthostatic blood pressure changes, and hypotension. In anorexia nervosa, this is primarily due to restriction of fluid intake, whereas in bulimia nervosa, self-induced vomiting and abuse of laxatives and diuretics are usually implicated.

A variety of cardiac conduction defects and rhythm disturbances are well described in patients with eating disorders (Brown and Mehler 2000). Indeed, sudden cardiac death is a leading cause of mortality in anorexia nervosa and bulimia nervosa. Electrolyte abnormalities are the major cause of serious rhythm disturbances and cardiac deaths in patients with eating disorders. Hypokalemia and, less frequently, hypocalcemia, hypophosphatemia, or hypomagnesemia predispose patients to potentially fatal ventricular arrhythmias.

Other cardiac complications of eating disorders are less common. Refeeding cardiomyopathy may result from overly aggressive refeeding in anorexia nervosa. Bulimics who abuse ipecac can develop ipecac-associated cardiomyopathy (Dresser et al. 1992). Because of the long half-life of ipecac, the drug can accumulate in cardiac tissue and cause prolonged or even irreversible cardiac dysfunction.

For an assessment of the potential cardiovascular complications, most patients with eating disorders should receive a baseline electrocardiogram. This is particularly important in low-weight patients with anorexia nervosa, patients with bulimia nervosa who are actively purging or abusing other medications, and patients with binge eating disorder who are obese. Electrocardiogram abnormalities in patients with eating disorders are of major concern; however, their true prevalence is somewhat controversial, ranging from very frequent in some studies to virtually nonexistent in others. However, serious abnormalities such as prolongation of the Q-T interval clearly do occur and predispose patients to potentially life-threatening arrhythmias. If significant abnormalities are identified, especially conduction defects, rhythm disturbances, or a prolonged Q-T interval, frequent monitoring of the electrocardiogram is indicated until normal weight is restored and/or cessation of bulimic behaviors has been achieved.

Mitral valve prolapse is reportedly common in patients with anorexia nervosa (Meyers et al. 1987), but the true prevalence and increased risk are difficult to discern because mitral valve prolapse is quite common in young women in the general population and well-matched control groups have not been included in many studies. If in fact echocardiographic evaluation for evidence of mitral valve prolapse is pursued more aggressively in patients with eating disorders, an artificially inflated frequency of diagnosis may result. Prolapse results from the decreased left ventricular size that accompanies dramatic weight loss, resulting in disproportion between the ventricle and the mitral valve. This abnormality appears to be reversible with weight gain.

Renal and Electrolytes

Electrolyte abnormalities are a major cause of morbidity and mortality in patients with eating disorders (Mitchell et al. 1983, 1987b), especially anorectic patients with major weight loss and bulimic patients engaging in severe purging and laxative or diuretic abuse. Many of the deaths attributable to eating disorders can be linked to hypokalemia. Low serum potassium levels may result from decreased intake and/or increased potassium losses due to self-induced vomiting or laxative or diuretic abuse. Careful monitoring of serum potassium levels in such patients throughout the course of treatment is a major responsibility of the clinician. Unfortunately, correction of hypokalemia can be quite difficult. Purging behaviors such as diuretic abuse and vomiting result in a hypochloremic contraction alkalosis that must be corrected before potassium supplements will prove effective. Hypokalemia, if persistent, can directly cause organ dysfunction. Cardiac arrhythmias and decreased cardiac performance are the most obvious consequences, but hypokalemic nephropathy and myopathy are also important. Hypokalemic nephropathy may be associated with elevated blood urea nitrogen and serum creatinine levels and even chronic renal failure.

Elevated blood urea nitrogen and creatinine levels may also reflect fluid depletion, hypovolemia, and decreased glomerular filtration rate (Boag et al. 1985). Fluid restriction may be a symptom of anorexia nervosa (Lowinger et al. 1999). Hypomagnesemia is not uncommon in anorectic patients and may be associated with persistent hypocalcemia or hypokalemia, which will resolve only if magnesium is replaced simultaneously. Hyperphosphatemia may be present in patients who vomit excessively. Conversely, profound hypophosphatemia can complicate refeeding and result in myocardial dysfunction and neurological complications, especially seizures (Wada et al. 1992).

Prolonged purging and/or diuretic or laxative abuse can result in a hypovolemic state that stimulates the renin-angiotensin-aldosterone system as homeostatic mechanisms attempt to conserve fluids (Mitchell et al. 1988b). When the patient attempts to curtail diuretic or laxative use, persistent hyperaldosteronism results in reflex edema formation. Unfortunately, this often triggers severe anxiety about weight gain and resumption of diuretic or laxative abuse. This self-perpetuating cycle can be extremely difficult to interrupt, and the patient must be reassured that fluid retention is a temporary condition that will resolve if bulimic behaviors can be avoided.

Endocrinologic

Amenorrhea is frequent in patients with anorexia nervosa, although the exact etiology remains incompletely defined (Devlin et al. 1989; Katz and Vollenhaven 2000). Amenorrhea may result from weight loss per se; cessation of menses is quite predictable in starvation from other causes.

However, menstruation has been reported to cease before any weight loss in some patients, and a history of irregular menses precedes the onset of anorexia in up to one-third of patients. Consequently, some authorities speculate that both amenorrhea and disordered eating may be attributable to a primary hypothalamic abnormality. Severe anorexia nervosa is associated with low levels of plasma estradiol, luteinizing hormone (LH), and follicle-stimulating hormone (FSH) (Brown and Mehler 2000). An "immature" response (resembling that of premenarchal girls) of LH and FSH to gonadotropin-releasing hormones is observed (Katz and Vollenhaven 2000). Generally speaking, these endocrine abnormalities normalize with successful weight gain, but there may be a significant lag period or persistent irregularities of menstrual function.

Menstrual abnormalities are also seen in patients with bulimia nervosa (Comerci 1990; deZwaan and Mitchell 1992; Pirke et al. 1987), although less frequently than in those with anorexia nervosa. In bulimia nervosa, a pattern of irregular menses is more common than amenorrhea. A decreased number of LH secretory spikes and abnormal LH responses to gonadotropin-releasing hormones have been reported in some bulimic patients.

Thyroid function test results are frequently abnormal in patients with anorexia nervosa (Thomas and Rebar 1990). The most common finding in anorectic patients is a normal T_4, decreased T_3, and normal thyroid-stimulating hormone (TSH). The "low T_3 syndrome" is due to decreased peripheral conversion of T_4 to T_3. There is preferential deiodination to "reverse T_3," a less active form of the hormone. The secretion of TSH is normal unless there is simultaneous thyroid gland failure. The response of TSH to provocative testing with exogenous thyroid-releasing hormone is intact but delayed. Anorectic patients frequently note symptoms of cold intolerance, and bradycardia, dry skin, and constipation are frequently observed. These represent a normal adaptation to starvation and the hypometabolic state and can be considered a physiologic response to low body weight. The most appropriate treatment for these patients is weight gain; thyroid hormone administration is not indicated for patients with "low T_3 syndrome" and a normal TSH. However, a few patients with eating disorders will coincidentally have true thyroid dysfunction. Because the symptoms of eating disorder and thyroid dysfunction are often similar, all patients with eating disorders should have their thyroid function tested.

Extensive abnormalities of the hypothalamic-pituitary-adrenal (HPA) system occur in anorexia nervosa (Boyar et al. 1977; Gold et al. 1986; Gwirtsman et al. 1989; Laue et al. 1991). Sustained hypercortisolism is a hallmark characteristic of anorexia nervosa. Both plasma and cerebrospinal levels of free cortisol are elevated. High cortisol levels have been attributed to both increased production and decreased metabolic clearance of the hormone. Nonsuppression of cortisol by dexamethasone is common in patients with anorexia nervosa. Plasma adrenocorticotropic hormone (ACTH) levels are generally normal, but cerebrospinal fluid ACTH levels have been reported to be low.

The HPA system has been less extensively evaluated in patients with bulimia nervosa (Gwirtsman et al. 1989; Hudson et al. 1983; Laue et al. 1991; Mortola et al. 1989). Most studies have found that plasma cortisol and ACTH levels in patients with bulimia are similar to those of control subjects. Others have reported that a subset of bulimic women, including some of normal weight, have elevated plasma cortisol and ACTH levels with blunted responses to corticotropin-releasing factor. Nonsuppression on the dexamethasone test occurs in some bulimic patients. Again, the etiology is unclear. Some abnormal dexamethasone suppression test (DST) results may be due to sustained hypercortisolism, whereas others may be due to erratic absorption of dexamethasone in bulimic patients with altered gastrointestinal function (Mitchell et al. 1984).

Studies of cortisol in patients with binge eating disorder are not available. However, it is known that obese patients, at least some of whom presumably binge eat, have abnormal DST results. This is usually due to inadequate dosage of dexamethasone in obese patients with a large volume of distribution. Repeat testing with 2 mg (instead of 1 mg) of dexamethasone will often result in normal suppression.

Anorexia nervosa is associated with impaired or erratic release of vasopressin. Many patients, therefore, develop partial neurogenic diabetes insipidus, characterized by polyuria and polydipsia. There is often a lag period after weight gain before these abnormalities reverse.

Other endocrine abnormalities in the eating disorders are less well documented. Acute hypoglycemia has been reported anecdotally (Rich et al. 1990). Prolactin levels are generally reported to be normal. One study found elevated serum prolactin values, whereas others have found decreased prolactin levels in patients with anorexia nervosa and some patients with bulimia nervosa (Kiriike et al. 1987). In anorexia nervosa, growth hormone may be elevated, as in other forms of starvation. Elevated basal levels of growth hormone probably reflect decreased production of somatomedin C. Some studies have demonstrated pathologic growth hormone responsiveness to provocative stimuli such as thyroid-releasing hormone or to glucose administration, but others have failed to confirm these results. Elevated growth hormone levels, promoting gluconeogenesis and reducing peripheral use of glucose, represent a protective physiologic adaptation to the state of starvation.

Gastrointestinal

Gastrointestinal complications are a prominent cause of morbidity for persons with eating disorders (Ceullar and VanThiel 1986; Crowell et al. 1993; McClain et al. 1993). Swelling of the parotid or submandibular glands is a classic finding in bulimia nervosa and is often one of the few physical examination clues to the diagnosis. Parotid hypertrophy may result in macroamylasemia; differentiation of hyperamylasemia secondary to pancreatitis by measuring amylase isoenzymes can be helpful. Parotid hypertrophy has also been described in malnourished patients with anorexia who do not purge (Kinzl et al. 1993; Mandel and Kaynar 1992). Resolution of parotid and salivary gland hypertrophy after successful treatment of the eating disorder is the norm, although this can take several months.

Abnormal gastrointestinal motility is a major problem for many patients with eating disorders (Anderson et al. 1997; Ceullar et al. 1988; Kamal et al. 1991). Impaired gastric emptying, described in patients with anorexia nervosa or bulimia nervosa, probably contributes to symptoms of bloating and early satiety. In most cases, treatment should be directed at management of the underlying eating disorder and reassurance of the patient. Altered gastrointestinal motility with prolonged whole-gut transit times has been well documented and may contribute to abdominal pain, constipation, and ileus. Patients with anorexia nervosa and constipation often have anorectal motor abnormalities (Chiarioni et al. 2000). Abnormal gut motility can be exacerbated by hypokalemic ileus or ileus secondary to superimposed pancreatitis. In anorexia nervosa, abdominal pain can also be due to compression of the third portion of the duodenum by the superior mesenteric artery (Adson et al. 1997).

Esophageal problems seen with eating disorders are diverse and range from mild esophagitis to esophageal rupture. Esophagitis, erosions, ulcerations, and bleeding are frequently observed in bulimic patients with recurrent self-induced vomiting. Mallory-Weiss tears may lead to significant gastrointestinal bleeding. Esophageal rupture (Boerhaave's syndrome) is a catastrophic manifestation requiring emergent medical and surgical intervention. Chronic sequelae of recurrent vomiting include the development of esophageal strictures or Barrett's esophagus.

Acute gastric dilatation and rupture have been described in bulimic patients during bingeing and in anorectic patients during refeeding (Abdu et al. 1987; Nakao et al. 2000). Rapid onset of nausea, vomiting, or abdominal pain may indicate gastric distention and in most cases can be treated conservatively by nasogastric suction and fluid and electrolyte replacement. In extreme cases, gastric rupture can occur, causing dramatic pain, sepsis, and shock and requiring emergent surgical intervention.

Colonic complications, especially constipation and abdominal pain, may be attributable to decreased oral intake, dehydration, or altered motility. Laxative abuse can cause or exacerbate these symptoms, because chronic use of stimulant laxatives may result in loss of normal peristaltic function. Laxative abusers usually complain of periods of diarrhea alternating with episodes of constipation. Cathartic colon can become severe and may even necessitate colonic resection. Chronic, recurrent use of laxatives may result in gastrointestinal bleeding, ranging from occult to frank blood loss. Long-term complications may also include malabsorption, steatorrhea, or protein-losing gastroenteropathy. Nonspecific inflammation or melanosis coli may be seen on colonoscopic examination.

Acute pancreatitis can develop during bingeing in patients with bulimia nervosa or during refeeding in those with anorexia nervosa, or because of associated alcohol abuse. Careful monitoring through abdominal examination is indicated in these patients. If signs or symptoms of pancreatitis, such as abdominal pain, nausea, or vomiting, are observed, measurement of serum amylase and isoenzymes will suggest the correct diagnosis. When pancreatitis is diagnosed, treatment with bowel rest, nasogastric suction, and intravenous fluid replacement should be promptly instituted.

Metabolic

Skeletal abnormalities are serious complications of anorexia nervosa (Biller et al. 1989; Brown and Mehler 2000; Jagielska et al. 2001; Newman and Halmi 1989; Rigotti et al. 1984; Salisbury and Mitchell 1991). Delayed bone maturation (chronological age greater than bone age), decreased bony density (osteoporosis), and pathologic fractures are consistently reported in patients with anorexia nervosa (Lucas et al. 1999). The extent of bone demineralization has generally been found to correlate with body mass index and duration of illness (Andersen 1992; Grinspoon et al. 1999).

The mechanism by which patients with anorexia nervosa develop osteoporosis is presumed to be multifactorial (Katz and Vollenhaven 2000; Lennkh et al. 1999; Newman and Halmi 1989). The low estrogen levels in these patients appear to be the major etiologic factor in the pathogenesis of osteoporosis, akin to the development of decreased bone mineral density in other estrogen-deficient states such as post-menopausal osteoporosis. However, nutritional factors also appear to contribute, because osteoporosis associated with anorexia nervosa is more severe than that seen in other low estrogen states (Grinspoon et al. 1999). The precise method by which hypogonadism causes bone loss remains to be determined. Reduced levels of the nutritionally dependent bone trophic factor IGF-1 appear to contribute to osteopenia in patients with anorexia nervosa (Soyka et al. 1999). However, disordered calcium regulation and bone remodeling, possibly mediated by estrogen effects on osteoclasts and osteoblasts or altered interleukin-6 levels, have been implicated. The sustained hypercortisolism observed in patients with anorexia nervosa may also play a role in the development of osteoporosis. Other factors such as decreased calcium intake, low vitamin D levels, or excess growth hormone may play less important roles in the etiology of osteoporosis in anorexia nervosa. In contrast, the excess exercise pursued by many patients with anorexia nervosa may actually have a protective effect. Osteoporosis is not usually seen in patients with bulimia nervosa unless they have a previous history of anorexia nervosa and low weight.

Other metabolic abnormalities have been reported in patents with anorexia nervosa and bulimia nervosa. Hypercholesterolemia is frequently observed in patients with anorexia nervosa, in contrast to other forms of starvation in which low serum cholesterol levels are expected. Elevated serum carotene levels are found in nearly three-fourths of patients with anorexia nervosa and may be associated with frank carotenodermia (Gupta et al. 1987). Hypercarotenemia is primarily a result of elevation of vitamin A active carotenoids, especially beta carotene. Zinc deficiency has been anecdotally reported in some patients with anorexia nervosa, and other trace metal and vitamin deficiencies such as pellagra and scurvy have on occasion been observed in patients with diet peculiarities.

The major medical complication of binge eating disorder is obesity. Obesity is a common problem in the industrialized world, affecting one-fourth of Americans. Morbid obesity, usually defined as weight greater than 170% of ideal body weight, affects about 3%–5% of the population. Obesity may be complicated by a variety of medical conditions, with the risk increasing as the degree of overweight increases (Table 7–4) (Atkinson 1991).

Cardiovascular complications are a major source of morbidity and mortality in obese individuals. Obese patients have an increased risk of hypertension and atherosclerotic cardiovascular disease, including myocardial infarction (Alpert and Hashimi 1993). In addition, the combination of hypertension and obesity may result in ventricular hypertrophy and eventually cardiomyopathy and heart failure (Benotti et al. 1992). Obese patients also have an increased incidence of cerebrovascular accidents.

Table 7–4. Medical complications of obesity

Cardiovascular	Hypertension Atherosclerotic cardiovascular disease; including myocardial infarction Ventricular hypertrophy and congestive heart failure Cerebrovascular accidents
Endocrine	Diabetes mellitus
Gastrointestinal	Gall bladder disease; risk further increased during rapid weight loss Fatty liver, portal inflammation and fibrosis—"nonalcoholic steatohepatitis"
Metabolic	Hyperlipidemia, especially hypertriglyceridemia Gout
Skeletal	Degenerative osteoarthritis
Pulmonary	Sleep apnea Obesity hypoventilation syndrome (Pickwickian syndrome)
Other	Increased cancer risk, especially breast, uterus, colon, prostate Increased surgical risk Decreased fertility (men and women) Adverse perinatal outcomes Early mortality

Overweight patients are at increased risk for several endocrine and metabolic conditions. Diabetes mellitus is frequently diagnosed in obese patients. The mechanism remains incompletely understood, but it is clear that insulin resistance is critical to the pathogenesis. Metabolic abnormalities in obesity, including hyperlipidemia, especially hypertriglyceridemia, undoubtedly contribute to accelerated development of atherosclerosis. An increased risk of gout also characterizes obesity.

Many gastrointestinal illnesses have been described in obese patients. Cholesterol gallstones are a recognized complication both of obesity and, paradoxically, of rapid weight loss (Shiffman et al. 1991). Gallstone disease occurs in about one-third of morbidly obese patients. Furthermore, gallstone formation has been reported to accompany rapid weight loss due to very-low-calorie diets or gastric bypass surgery in up to one-fourth of patients (Worobetz et al. 1993). Gallstones will resolve spontaneously in about half of these patients, but symptoms will necessitate cholecystectomy in the remainder. Abnormal liver enzymes (especially lactate dehydrogenase and serum transaminases) usually reflect fatty infiltration of the liver in obese patients (Andersen 1992). Portal inflammation and fibrosis, called "nonalcoholic steatohepatitis," also occurs in many of the massively obese.

Obese patients frequently have a variety of musculoskeletal complaints. These probably relate primarily to the high incidence of degenerative osteoarthritis seen in obesity. Wear and tear on joints such as the knees is directly attributable to the excess stress placed on weight-bearing joints in the obese.

Obesity causes chronic airflow limitation with decreased lung capacities, even in nonsmokers (Rubinstein et al. 1991; Sugarman et al. 1992). In the most severe cases, respiratory insufficiency, commonly known as Pickwickian syndrome, may develop. Obese patients may develop obstructive sleep apnea syndrome or obesity hypoventilation syndrome. In sleep apnea, the patient experiences intermittent pauses in breathing, especially while sleeping, resulting in hypoxia, disrupted sleep, and daytime somnolence. Excessive snoring is a major clue to sleep apnea. In contrast, obesity hypoventilation syndrome results in hypoxia at any time and is due to decreased lung volumes. Long-term complications of these syndromes include pulmonary hypertension, arrhythmias, cardiac failure, and increased risk of sudden death (Rajala et al. 1991; Rossner et al. 1991).

Other medical complications of obesity include an increased risk of cancer, especially of the breast, uterus, colon, or prostate; increased surgical risk, including postoperative pneumonias, wound infections, and deep venous thrombosis; and increased mortality. Decreased fertility is common in the obese, with abnormal menstrual function in women and abnormal sperm production in men. An increased risk of adverse perinatal outcomes has been reported for obese women (Perlow et al. 1992).

Pulmonary

Bulimic patients with recurrent vomiting are at risk of developing aspiration pneumonia or chemical pneumonitis secondary to inhalation of gastric acid. In addition, spontaneous pneumothorax, pneumomediastinum, and subcutaneous emphysema can occur in patients with anorexia nervosa or bulimia nervosa. The mechanism is poorly studied, but it seems logical that vomiting could raise intrathoracic pressures and rupture a bleb or other weakened area of the lung. However, this complication has been described in anorectic patients who do not vomit, possibly secondary to poor tissue integrity due to malnutrition. Ventilatory failure, presumably caused by a combination of decreased energy reserves and electrolyte abnormalities, has been reported in severe cases of anorexia nervosa (Ryan et al. 1992).

Dermatologic

The dermatologic manifestations of eating disorders have been classified into four subgroups: 1) complications associated with starvation and malnutrition, 2) complications of self-induced vomiting, 3) complications of abuse of laxatives, diuretics, or ipecac, and 4) complications associated with concomitant psychiatric illness (Gupta et al. 1987).

Nearly one-third of patients with anorexia nervosa will develop increased lanugo-like hair on the face and other parts of the body. This may be accompanied by loss of scalp hair. Dry scaly skin and brittle hair and nails are common in anorexia nervosa. Hypercarotenemia and carotenodermia may be present in patients with anorexia nervosa, in contradistinction to other forms of starvation. Rare cases of pellagra (niacin deficiency) or scurvy (vitamin C deficiency) may be associated with the skin changes characteristic of these deficiencies. Rarely, petechiae or purpura may be clues to thrombocytopenia resulting from starvation-induced hypoplasia of bone marrow.

Calluses, abrasions, and/or bruising of the dorsum of the hand or thumb, called "Russell's sign," are the classic clue to the recurrent self-induced vomiting characteristic of bulimia nervosa. Damage to the skin is caused by rubbing of the fingers or thumb against the teeth during induction of vomiting by manual stimulation of the gag reflex. Transient facial purpura or conjunctival hemorrhage may result from the increased intrathoracic pressures generated during recurrent vomiting.

Fixed drug eruptions, such as photosensitivity due to thiazide diuretics, are dermatologic clues to the abuse of drugs consumed to lose weight. Finally, self-induced dermatoses from repetitive excoriation of the skin, compulsive hand-washing, or trichotillomania have been reported in patients with eating disorders and comorbid psychiatric conditions.

Hematologic/Immunologic

Leukopenia, anemia, and thrombocytopenia have been reported in persons with anorexia nervosa (Howard et al. 1992). If starvation is severe, frank bone marrow necrosis can occur (Bailly et al. 1994; Smith and Spivak 1985). Leukopenia usually reflects decreased neutrophil numbers; relative lymphocytosis is the norm, but total lymphocyte counts may be decreased. Low white cell counts do not appear to increase risk of infection, possibly because bone marrow neutrophil reserves are normal (Bowers and Eckert 1978), but this is controversial (Devuyst et al. 1993) and further study is needed. Neutrophils may also have disordered functional capacity. Abnormalities of chemotaxis and microbicidal activity have been reported, but not in all anorectic patients or in all studies. Significant reductions in complement, especially components of the alternative pathway, have been described (Pomeroy et al. 1997). Immunoglobulin levels have been reported to be low in some patients with anorexia nervosa, but these findings have been refuted by others.

Lymphocyte phenotypes in patients with anorexia nervosa have been the subject of several studies, with varying results. Some authors report that $CD4^+$ cells are normal, whereas others have found decreased $CD4^+$ counts as observed in other forms of starvation. Low $CD8^+$ counts have been described (Fink et al. 1996). Delayed type hypersensitivity skin testing is an excellent screening test for responsivity of the immune system, especially cell-mediated immunity. Failure to respond to skin testing (anergy) is characteristic of patients with anorexia nervosa who weigh less than 60% of ideal body weight. Variable responses are obtained when the patient has less severe weight loss.

Despite suggestions of multiple perturbations of immune function in anorexia nervosa, it appears that these patients remain remarkably free of infections (Bowers and Eckert 1978). Exploration of this apparent paradox requires additional investigation. Recent investigations have focused on a possible role of cytokines in the ability to resist infection, as well as a more general role in the pathogenesis of anorexia nervosa and/or its associated medical complications. Cytokines are polypeptides that act as molecular signals for communications between cells, especially cells of the immune, neurologic, and endocrine systems. In some cases, tumor necrosis factor–α, interleukin-6, and transforming growth factor–β were elevated in patients with untreated anorexia nervosa and normalized with refeeding (Pomeroy et al. 1994). In contrast, in other studies, production of interleukin-1, interleukin-6, and tumor necrosis factor–α was decreased in anorexia nervosa and recovered only with the start of weight gain (Nagata et al. 1999). Further studies are needed to determine the pathophysiologic significance of these findings.

Neurologic

Because many of the basic control systems for feeding behavior and neuroendocrine function are located in the central nervous system, examination of the neurological system has been an area of research emphasis in the eating disorders (Krieg et al. 1987, 1988, 1989). A variety of structural abnormalities of the brain have been described in patients with anorexia and have been linked to cognitive dysfunction (Katzman et al. 2001). Computed tomography scans demonstrate enlarged ventricles and external cerebrospinal fluid spaces in many patients with anorexia nervosa and some patients with bulimia nervosa (Herholz 1996). These abnormalities have been termed "pseudoatrophy" of the brain because they generally normalize after weight gain (Addolorato et al. 1998).

Positron emission tomography has been used to study brain function in patients with anorexia nervosa (Herholz et al. 1987). Abnormal glucose metabolism has been noted in these patients during starvation. These findings again raise the possibility of primary central nervous system dysfunction in patients with eating disorders, but this remains speculative.

Dental

Dental complications are generally confined to the subset of patients with eating disorders who engage in repetitive, self-induced vomiting (Milosevic 1999; Milosevic et al. 1997; Roberts and Li 1987; Simmons et al. 1986; Studen-Pavlovich and Elliott 2001). Decalcification of the lingual, palatal, and posterior occlusive surfaces of the teeth is referred to as *perimylolysis* and results from erosion by gastric acid during vomiting. Because amalgams are resistant to acid, they become much more obvious as enamel erosion progresses. Increased temperature sensitivity and increased incidence of caries have also been reported but not confirmed in all studies. Involvement of a concerned dentist and careful dental examinations are a critical component of treatment for patients with bulimia nervosa and patients with anorexia nervosa who vomit.

Temperature Regulation

Disordered thermoregulation is a common complaint of patients with eating disorders. Persons with anorexia nervosa often demonstrate aberrant autonomic responses when exposed to extremes of environmental temperature. In one study, thermal sweating was observed to occur at lower core and skin temperatures in patients with anorexia nervosa than in control subjects. Some patients with eating disorders also complain of Raynaud's phenomenon in the cold and easy vasodilatation and swelling of the hands and feet in warm temperatures. It has been proposed that some anorectic patients have a central thermoregulatory disorder, possibly another manifestation of hypothalamic dysfunction. Symptoms of disordered thermoregulation can be quite distressing to the patient, but no specific therapy is available.

ABUSE OF LAXATIVES, DIURETICS, DIET PILLS, AND IPECAC

Individuals with eating disorders may misuse a variety of drugs in an attempt to promote weight loss by suppressing appetite, minimizing food absorption, eliminating fluid, or inducing vomiting (Mitchell and Boutacoff 1986; Mitchell et al. 1985, 1987a, 1987b). Persons with bulimia may abuse laxatives, diuretics, diet pills, and/or ipecac. It is estimated that nearly two-thirds use laxatives and one-third use diuretics in attempts to augment weight loss.

Laxatives

Some patients with bulimia nervosa ingest huge amounts of laxative drugs, many times in excess of the amount recommended by the manufacturer (Mitchell and Boutacoff 1986; Mitchell et al. 1988a; Turner et al. 2000). Stimulant-type laxatives are most frequently used and are available in many over-the-counter preparations. Abuse of laxatives is not an effective method of weight reduction, because laxative-induced weight loss occurs predominantly due to transient loss of fluids or stool rather than prevention of calorie absorption. Furthermore, laxative use precipitates activation of the renin-angiotensin-aldosterone system, and secondary hyperaldosteronism subsequently promotes fluid retention. Chronic use of laxatives can result in serious sequelae, including loss of the normal colonic peristalsis (laxative dependency) and cathartic colon (loss of normal colon function). This results in a potentially vicious cycle of further laxative abuse. It has been recognized that bulimics may also use enemas in an attempt to lose weight (Mitchell et al. 1991). Fleet enemas or tap water enemas may be used as often as several times a week or daily.

Diuretics

Diuretics are available in a wide variety of over-the-counter formulations for treatment of premenstrual symptoms and are frequently used in large quantities by patients with bulimia nervosa to promote weight loss (Mitchell et al. 1988a; Pomeroy and Mitchell 1989). Pamabrom is the main active ingredient in many of the currently available over-the-counter diuretic preparations. Diuretic use may begin as an attempt to control "edema" and progress to abuse, with ingestion of diuretics in progressively larger quantities over time. Indeed, the initial diuretic use may promote secondary hyperaldosteronism and reflex fluid retention when diuretics are discontinued. Instead of allowing the system to readjust and fluid balance to be restored, the patient resumes diuretic use believing that continued diuretic use is required to control the edema.

Patients with bulimia nervosa may also abuse prescription diuretics. This is particularly common among health care workers who have access to such medications. Thiazide diuretics such as hydrochlorothiazide, loop diuretics such as furosemide, and potassium-sparing diuretics such as spironolactone and triamterene have all been described as drugs of abuse in bulimia nervosa. Physicians should exercise caution in prescribing these medications for at-risk individuals, especially if the reason for the drug request is vague or poorly documented.

Diet Pills

Phenylpropanolamine is the active ingredient in most over-the-counter diet pills. Although many individuals with eating disorders use diet pills at some point in the course of their illness, long-term, high-dose abuse is uncommon, possibly because of the untoward side effects of these drugs or their relative lack of effectiveness in promoting weight loss. However, abuse of over-the-counter diet pills, either alone or in combination with illicit amphetamines, has been well documented. In addition, some patients may abuse thyroid hormone in an attempt to induce a hypermetabolic state and weight loss. Abuse of any of these agents may result in anxiety and agitation as well as hypertension and seizures in some patients and may even precipitate strokes or intracranial hemorrhage in susceptible individuals. These drugs should never be ingested in amounts in excess of the manufacturers' recommendations, and the patient should have close medical follow-up while they are being used.

Ipecac

Although ipecac has undoubtedly saved lives, it has emerged as a serious drug of abuse in patients with eating disorders (Mitchell et al. 1988a; Palmer and Guay 1985). Huge quantities of ipecac may be repetitively ingested to induce vomiting. The active ingredient, emetine, has a long half-life, resulting in accumulation of large amounts of drug in the body over time. Serious skeletal muscle myopathy and cardiomyopathy can result. Recovery may be prolonged, and fatalities due to ipecac-induced cardiomyopathy have been reported.

MANAGEMENT OF MEDICAL COMPLICATIONS OF EATING DISORDERS

Nutritional management is obviously a critical component of therapy for patients with an eating disorder (American Dietetic Association 2001). Many different regimens for refeeding the patient with anorexia nervosa have been successfully used (Becker et al. 1999). A combination of supportive nursing care and behavioral techniques is usually most effective (Kaye et al. 1999). In general, nasogastric tube feeding or hyperalimentation are indicated only for patients with severe weight loss that has been refractory to the usual therapeutic modalities. An expected weight gain of 1–2 lb/week is generally considered optimal. More rapid caloric replacement can result in serious medical complications, including electrolyte abnormalities and refeeding pancreatitis or cardiomyopathy. For patients with bulimia nervosa and those who binge eat, reinforcement of normal eating behaviors is the goal (McGilley and Pryor 1998). Both psychological interventions—especially cognitive behavioral therapy—and pharmacological treatment with antidepressants may be effective (Kaye et al. 1999; Wilfley and Cohen 1997). All health care providers should be actively involved in emphasizing the medical need for good eating habits.

The best methods for voluntary weight loss and control remain incompletely studied and controversial (National Institutes of Health Technology Assessment Conference Panel 1992). Multiple methodologies including meal planning, support groups, and intensive behavioral approaches may be useful (Arrone 1998; Barlow and Dietz 1998; National Institutes of Health 1998), but often are rewarded with only transient effects. Other approaches, such as surgery and very-low-calorie diets, require more intensive medical monitoring and should be reserved for severe cases. Surgical approaches to weight reduction have been associated with significant medical risks. After jejunoileal bypass, up to 6% of patients develop gallstones and, more importantly, liver injury occurs in about 3% of patients, with a 20% fatality rate. As a result, this procedure has been largely supplanted by gastric bypass or gastroplasty. Liver injury and gallstones are complications of these newer procedures as well, albeit at a lower rate. Thus, surgical approaches should be limited to those patients with potentially life-threatening complications of obesity (such as sleep apnea) in whom nonsurgical therapies have failed.

Early use of liquid protein diets proved to have a variety of untoward consequences, especially electrolyte disturbances, cardiac arrhythmias, and sudden death. Very-low-calorie diets in more recent formulations can be safe if used as directed and with careful medical supervision

(Anderson et al. 1992; Pi-Sunyer 1992; Seim et al. 1995). Nevertheless, patients must be closely monitored, especially for complications such as gallstone formation.

For many patients with eating disorders, electrolyte abnormalities are the most prominent medical complication. The medical clinician should closely follow these patients to ensure adequate correction of electrolyte values. Asymptomatic hypokalemia should generally be treated with oral potassium supplementation; intravenous replacement should be reserved for hospitalized patients with very low potassium levels or patients with symptoms attributable to hypokalemia. There are no absolute guidelines for when to institute potassium replacement; treatment decisions must be individualized based on severity of electrolyte abnormalities, chronicity, and anticipated compliance. It is often reasonable to begin oral potassium supplements when the serum potassium falls below 3.2–3.3 mEq/L (normal range 3.5–5.0 mEq/L) and to consider hospitalization if potassium levels are below 2.8–3.0 mEq/L. However, it must be emphasized that no level is "safe," and the level of serum potassium cannot be reliably used to predict when complications will occur in an individual patient. Unfortunately, many patients with eating disorders are reluctant to comply with oral potassium replacement regimens; careful explanation of the importance of the intervention is critical. The efficacy of potassium supplements is often attenuated by the presence of contraction metabolic alkalosis. The patient must understand that cessation of vomiting is necessary if treatment is to be successful. In the presence of severe electrolyte abnormalities, hospitalization for intravenous fluid and electrolyte management may be life saving.

Treatment of hypogonadism, with its attendant complications of amenorrhea and osteoporosis, has been inadequately studied, and conclusive recommendations cannot be made at this time (Kreipe and Mou 2000). Nevertheless, osteoporosis and the risk of pathologic fractures are a major concern in most anorectic and some bulimic patients. Some authors have suggested that cyclic estrogen replacement (with or without progesterone) and/or oral calcium supplementation should be used to maintain or restore bone mineral density, but this is controversial (Bruni et al. 2000; Robinson et al. 2000). Until results from controlled trials are available, the clinician will have to individualize this treatment decision (Ward et al. 1997). Obviously, these interventions are less desirable than treatment of the eating disorder and normalization of endocrine function by weight gain.

Frequent dental evaluation is strongly recommended for all patients who engage in recurrent vomiting (Hazelton and Faine 1996; Milosevic 1999; Milosevic et al. 1997). The use of bicarbonate rinses after vomiting may curtail enamel erosion. It remains unclear if brushing immediately after vomiting is beneficial or harmful; studies are ongoing (Milosevic et al. 1997). Patients with bulimia should be advised to use fluoridated mouth rinses daily and, if they continue to vomit, to rinse their mouths with bicarbonate rinses shortly after vomiting. Dentists caring for patients with bulimia nervosa should consider prescribing topical fluoride treatments. Careful dental evaluation is indicated on a frequent basis for all bulimic patients who engage in recurrent vomiting.

The importance of counseling patients to cease laxative, diuretic, diet pill, and ipecac abuse cannot be overemphasized. Attempts to discontinue these associated behaviors may be quite distressful to patients with eating disorders, and close follow-up during these periods is important. Patients who discontinue laxatives after chronic use often suffer from transient constipation. Resumption of stimulant laxatives should be avoided. Use of bulk-type laxatives, increased roughage in the diet, maintenance of normal hydration, and regular exercise can be used to assist with restoration of normal bowel function. Discontinuation of diuretics may also be quite difficult for patients. Because chronic diuretic use results in secondary hyperaldosteronism, patients may develop reflex edema when they attempt to stop taking diuretics, and reassurance that the fluid balance will soon normalize can be useful.

The medical clinician should collaborate with the eating disorder specialist to determine whether the patient with an eating disorder requires hospitalization. Obviously, medical emergencies such as cardiac arrhythmias, serious electrolyte disturbances, or significant gastrointestinal bleeding require admission and stabilization on a medical ward. Otherwise, the decision to hospitalize a patient for treatment of the eating disorder should be prompted by poor prognostic medical, psychiatric, or social factors. Specifically, hospitalization should be considered if a patient with anorexia has weight loss greater than 25%–30% of ideal body weight or a rapidly decreasing weight. Patients who are judged to be at significant risk of suicide or who have other serious comorbid psychiatric conditions such as intractable depression may also benefit from hospitalization. A poor social situation that will interfere with successful outpatient treatment of the eating disorder may also necessitate hospitalization. Finally, failure of intensive outpatient therapy may appropriately prompt admission to an inpatient facility.

Careful ongoing medical management is an essential component of the treatment plan for patients with eating disorders, and medical follow-up on a regular basis should be part of the treatment plan (Mehler 2001; Walsh et al. 2000). Frequency and content of medical visits must be individualized for each patient, depending on the severity and chronicity of the eating disorder and the associated medical complications. For medically stable patients, return visits approximately every 3 months may be appropriate and should include an interim history, focused physical examination, and laboratory testing. Follow-up evaluations should be done more frequently if medical complications have been identified, the patient's condition has deteriorated, or medical interventions are planned.

INTERACTIONS WITH OTHER MEDICAL CONDITIONS

Many medical diseases can be exacerbated by an eating disorder. Illnesses that require dietary control, such as hyperlipidemia, pancreatitis, malabsorption, or renal failure, can be very difficult to treat in patients with eating disorders. Supportive nutritional counseling by a nonjudgmental dietitian or other health care provider is required. The patient needs to understand that calorie restriction, binge eating, or purging behaviors can create a variety of nutritional imbalances that may adversely affect the course and outcome of the underlying medical illness.

Diabetes Mellitus

The patient with concurrent diabetes mellitus and an eating disorder presents a serious challenge to the clinician treating either condition (Rodin and Daneman 1992; Ward et al. 1995). Whether a specific association exists between these two disorders remains controversial, but it seems reasonable to speculate that certain aspects of diabetes and its treatment may trigger the expression of an eating disorder in susceptible individuals. Furthermore, management of diabetes is clearly complicated by the simultaneous presence of an eating disorder.

Control of diabetes obviously requires strict dietary management. The anorectic patient may be unwilling to comply with the specified caloric intake required to main good nutrition. Bulimic binge–purge behaviors make consistent control of glucose levels extremely difficult. Patients with eating disorders may provide inaccurate reports of their dietary intake. Perhaps of most concern, patients may withhold insulin in a deliberate attempt to induce glycosuria and subsequent weight loss. Such behaviors may contribute to impaired metabolic control with the attendant risks of hypoglycemia or diabetic ketoacidosis and may accelerate the development of the long-term microvascular complications of diabetes (Rydall et al. 1997).

The eating disorder patient with insulin-dependent diabetes requires the consistent support of a physician who understands that difficulties with body image are often exacerbated by concurrent diabetes. Both illnesses often result in a sense of lack of control, especially in adolescent patients. The endocrinologist and the eating disorder specialist must work together to ensure successful treatment for these patients.

Pregnancy

Infertility may result from an untreated eating disorder (Katz and Vollenhaven 2000; Stewart 1992). Recent studies have emphasized that eating disorders should be considered as an etiology of infertility and that screening for an eating disorder may obviate the need for expensive and uncomfortable gynecologic evaluations. Bulimic as well as anorectic patients may develop infertility as a complication of their eating disorder (Morgan 1999).

Pregnancy may be quite problematic for women with eating disorders (Katz and Vollenhaven 2000; Morgan et al. 1999). Discomfort with body image is often exacerbated by the physiologic changes that occur during pregnancy. This may worsen the severity of the pregnant woman's eating disorder, resulting in enhanced calorie restriction in anorexia nervosa and increased binge–purge episodes in bulimia nervosa (Franko and Spurrell 2000). Women with eating disorders seem to be at significantly increased risk of developing hyperemesis gravidarum (Katz and Vollenhaven 2000). Maternal weight gain is often inadequate in patients with a simultaneous eating disorder. Women who have an active eating disorder at the time of conception tend to have smaller babies with lower Apgar scores. Pregnant women with eating disorders may be at greater risk for delivery by cesarean section and for postpartum depression (Franko et al. 2001). They may also have greater difficulty with breastfeeding after delivery. A variety of other complications have been anecdotally described in pregnant women with eating disorders, including difficult labor, increased need for cesarean section, and increased risk of developing pregnancy-associated hypertension.

Authorities have recommended that a dietary review and a history of eating disorders be part of the routine assessment of patients with infertility problems, prenatal patients with hyperemesis gravidarum, and women who fail to gain weight adequately in pregnancy or who have small babies for gestational age (Franko and Spurrell 2000; Katz and Vollenhaven 2000). It may be advisable to suggest postponing pregnancy until the eating disorder is in remission (Katz and Vollenhaven 2000). If a woman with an eating disorder does become pregnant, careful collaboration between the obstetrician and eating disorder specialist is advisable to ensure the best outcome for the patient and her baby.

SUMMARY

Patients with eating disorders can develop multiple medical complications. Mental health care providers must be aware of the potentially serious nature of these complications, especially among patients who have anorexia nervosa, severe purging behaviors, or markedly abnormal body weight. Careful medical evaluation and ongoing medical management to prevent and treat potential medical complications are critical components in the care of such patients. Attention to medical complications is therefore an integral part of the comprehensive treatment plan for patients with eating disorders.

REFERENCES

Abdu RA, Garritano D, Culver O: Acute gastric necrosis in anorexia nervosa and bulimia. Arch Surg 122:830–832, 1987

Addolorato G, Taronto C, Capristo E, et al: A case of marked cerebellar atrophy in a women with anorexia nervosa and a review of the literature. Int J Eat Disord 24:443–447, 1998

Adson DE, Mitchell JE, Trenkner SW: The superior mesenteric artery syndrome and acute gastric dilatation in eating disorders: a report of two cases and a review of the literature. Int J Eat Disord 21:103–114, 1997

Agras WS: The consequences and costs of the eating disorders. Psychiatr Clin North Am 24:371–379, 2001

Alpert MA, Hashimi MW: Obesity and the heart. Am J Med Sci 306:117–123, 1993

American Dietetic Association: Position of the American Dietetic Association: nutrition intervention in the treatment of anorexia nervosa, bulimia nervosa, and eating disorders not otherwise specified (EDNOS). J Am Diet Assoc 101:810–819, 2001

Andersen T: Liver and gallbladder disease before and after very-low-calorie diets. Am J Clin Nutr 56:235–239, 1992

Anderson JW, Hamilton CC, Kaplan-Brinkman V: Benefits and risks of an intensive very-low-calorie diet program for severe obesity. Am J Gastroenterol 87:6–15, 1992

Anderson L, Shaw JM, McCargar L: Physiological effects of bulimia on the gastrointestinal tract. Can J Gastroenterol 11:451–459, 1997

Aronne LJ: Modern medical management of obesity: the role of pharmaceutical intervention. J Am Diet Assoc 98:523–526, 1998

Atkinson RL: Massive obesity: complications and treatment. Nutr Rev 49:49–53, 1991

Bailly D, Lambin I, Garzon G, et al: Bone marrow hypoplasia in anorexia nervosa: a case report. Int J Eat Disord 16:97–100, 1994

Barlow SE, Dietz WH: Obesity evaluation and treatment. Pediatrics 102:E29, 1998

Becker AE, Grinspoon SK, Klibanski A, et al: Eating disorders. N Engl J Med 340:1092–1098, 1999

Benotti PN, Bistrian B, Benotti JR, et al: Heart disease and hypertension in severe obesity: the benefits of weight reduction. Am J Clin Nutr 55:586–590, 1992

Biller BM, Saxe V, Herzog DB, et al: Mechanisms of osteoporosis in adult and adolescent women with anorexia nervosa. J Clin Endocrinol Metab 68:548–554, 1989

Boag F, Weerakoon J, Ginsburg J, et al: Diminished creatinine clearance in anorexia nervosa: reversal with weight gain. J Clin Pathol 38:60–63, 1985

Bowers TK, Eckert E: Leukopenia in anorexia nervosa: lack of increased risk of infection. Arch Intern Med 138:1520–1523, 1978

Boyar RM, Hellman KL, Roffwarg HP, et al: Cortisol secretion and metabolism in anorexia nervosa. N Engl J Med 296:190–193, 1977

Brown JM, Mehler PS: Medical complications occurring in adolescents with anorexia nervosa. West J Med 172:189–193, 2000

Bruce B, Wilfley D: Binge eating among the overweight population: a serious and prevalent problem. J Am Diet Assoc 96:58–61, 1996

Bruni V, Dei M, Vicini I, et al: Estrogen replacement therapy in the management of osteopenia related to eating disorders. Ann N Y Acad Sci 900:416–421, 2000

Ceullar RE, VanThiel DH: Gastrointestinal consequences of the eating disorders: anorexia nervosa and bulimia. Am J Gastroenterol 81:1113–1124, 1986

Ceullar RE, Kaye WH, Hsu LK, et al: Upper gastrointestinal tract dysfunction in bulimia. Dig Dis Sci 33:1549–1553, 1988

Chiarioni G, Bassotti G, Monsignori A, et al: Anorectal dysfunction in constipated women with anorexia nervosa. Mayo Clin Proc 75:1015–1019, 2000

Comerci G: Medical complications of anorexia nervosa and bulimia. Med Clin North Am 74:1293–1310, 1990

Cooke RA, Chambers JB: Anorexia nervosa and the heart. British Journal of Hospital Medicine 54:313–317, 1995

Crisp AH, Callender JS, Halek C, et al: Long-term mortality in anorexia nervosa. Br J Psychiatry 161:104–107, 1992

Crowell MD, Cheskin LJ, Musial F: Prevalence of gastrointestinal symptoms in obese and normal weight binge eaters. Am J Gastroenterol 89:387–391, 1993

Devlin MJ, Walsh BT, Katz JL, et al: Hypothalamic-pituitary-gonadal function in anorexia nervosa and bulimia. Psychiatry Res 28:11–24, 1989

Devuyst O, Lambert M, Rodhain J, et al: Hematological changes and infectious complications in anorexia nervosa: a case study. QJM 86:791–799, 1993

deZwaan M, Mitchell JE: Binge eating in the obese. Ann Med 24:303–308, 1992

Dresser LP, Massey EW, Johnson EE, et al: Ipecac myopathy and cardiomyopathy. J Neurol Neurosurg Psychiatry 55:560–562, 1992

Emborg C: Mortality and causes of death in eating disorders in Denmark 1970–1993: a case register study. Int J Eat Disord 25:243–251, 1999

Fichter MM, Quadflieg N: Six-year course and outcome of anorexia nervosa. Int J Eat Disord 26:359–385, 1999

Fink S, Eckert E, Mitchell J, et al: *t*-Lymphocyte subsets in patients with abnormal body weight: longitudinal studies in anorexia nervosa and obesity. Int J Eat Disorder 20:295–305, 1996

Franko DL, Spurrell EB: Detection and management of eating disorders during pregnancy. Obstet Gynecol 95:942–946, 2000

Franko DL, Blais MA, Becker AE, et al: Pregnancy complications and neonatal outcomes in women with eating disorders. Am J Psychiatry 158:1461–1466, 2001

Gold PW, Gwirtsman H, Avgerinos PC, et al: Abnormal hypothalamic-pituitary-adrenal function in anorexia nervosa. N Engl J Med 314:1335–1342, 1986

Grinspoon S, Miller K, Coyle C, et al: Severity of osteopenia in estrogen deficient women with anorexia nervosa and hypothalamic amenorrhea. J Clin Endocrinol Metab 84:2049–2055, 1999

Gupta MA, Gupta AK, Haberman HF: Dermatologic signs in anorexia nervosa and bulimia nervosa. Arch Dermatol 123:1386–1390, 1987

Gwirtsman HE, Kaye WH, George DT, et al: Central and peripheral ACTH and cortisol levels in anorexia nervosa and bulimia. Arch Gen Psychiatry 46:61–69, 1989

Hazelton LR, Faine MP: Diagnosis and dental management of eating disorder patients. Int J Prosthodont 9:65–73, 1996

Herholz K: Neuroimaging in anorexia nervosa. Psychiatry Res 62:105–110, 1996

Herholz K, Krieg JC, Emrich HM, et al: Regional cerebral glucose metabolism in anorexia nervosa measured by positron emission tomography. Biol Psychiatry 22:43–51, 1987

Herzog W, Deter H-C, Fiehn W, et al: Medical findings and predictors of long-term physical outcome in anorexia nervosa. Psychol Med 27:269–279, 1997

Howard MR, Leggat HM, Chaudhry S: Hematological and immunological abnormalities in eating disorders. Br J Hosp Med 48:234–239, 1992

Hudson J, Pope HG Jr, Jonas JM, et al: Hypothalamic-pituitary-adrenal axis hyperactivity in bulimia. Psychiatry 8:111–117, 1983

Isner JM, Roberts WC, Heymsfield SB, et al: Anorexia nervosa and sudden death. Ann Intern Med 102:49–52, 1985

Jagielska G, Wolanczyk T, Komender J, et al: Bone mineral content and bone mineral density in adolescent girls with anorexia nervosa: a longitudinal study. Acta Psychiatr Scand 104:131–137, 2001

Kamal N, Chami T, Andersen A, et al: Delayed gastrointestinal transit times in anorexia nervosa and bulimia nervosa. Gastroenterology 101:1320–1324, 1991

Katz MG, Vollenhaven B: The reproductive consequences of anorexia nervosa. Br J Obstet Gynecol 107:707–713, 2000

Katzman DK, Christensen B, Young AR, et al: Starving the brain: structural abnormalities and cognitive impairment in adolescents with anorexia nervosa. Semin Clin Neuropsychiatry 6:146–152, 2001

Kaye W, Strober M, Stein D, et al: New directions in treatment research of anorexia and bulimia nervosa. Biol Psychiatry 45:1285–1292, 1999

Kinzl J, Biebl W, Herold M: Significance of vomiting for hyperamylasemia and sialadenosis in patients with eating disorders. Int J Eat Disord 13:117–124, 1993

Kiriike N, Nishiwaki S, Izumiya Y, et al: Thyrotropin, prolactin, and growth hormone responses to thyrotropin-releasing hormone in anorexia nervosa and bulimia. Biol Psychiatry 22:167–176, 1987

Kreipe RE, Harris JP: Myocardial impairment resulting from eating disorders. Pediatr Ann 21:760–768, 1992

Kreipe RE, Mou SM: Eating disorders in adolescents and young adults. Obstet Gynecol Clin North Am 27:101–124, 2000

Krieg JC, Backmund H, Pirke KM: Cranial computed tomography findings in bulimia. Acta Psychiatr Scand 75:144–149, 1987

Krieg JC, Pirke KM, Lauer C, et al: Endocrine, metabolic, and cranial computed tomography findings in anorexia nervosa. Biol Psychiatry 23:377–387, 1988

Krieg JC, Lauer C, Leinsinger G, et al: Brain morphology and regional cerebral blood flow in anorexia nervosa. Biol Psychiatry 25:1041–1048, 1989

Laue L, Gold PW, Richmond A, et al: The hypothalamic-pituitary-adrenal axis in anorexia nervosa and bulimia nervosa: pathophysiologic implications. Adv Pediatr 38:287–316, 1991

Lennkh C, de Zwaan M, Bailer U, et al: Osteopenia in anorexia nervosa: specific mechanisms of bone loss. J Psychiatr Res 33:349–356, 1999

Lowinger K, Griffiths RA, Beumont PJ, et al: Fluid restriction in anorexia nervosa: a neglected symptom or new phenomenon? Int J Eat Disord 26:392–396, 1999

Lucas AR, Melton J, Crowson CS, et al: Long-term fracture risk among women with anorexia nervosa. Mayo Clin Proc 74:972–977, 1999

Mandel L, Kaynar A: Bulimia and parotid swelling: a review and case report. J Oral Maxillofac Surg 50:1122–1125, 1992

McClain C, Humphries LL, Hill KK, et al: Gastrointestinal and nutritional aspects of eating disorders. J Am Coll Nutr 12:466–474, 1993

McGilley BM, Pryor TL: Assessment and treatment of bulimia nervosa. Am Fam Physician 57:2743–2750, 1998

Mehler PS: Eating disorders, 1: anorexia nervosa. Hosp Pract 15:109–117, 1996a

Mehler PS: Eating disorders, 2: bulimia nervosa. Hosp Pract 15:107–126, 1996b

Mehler PS: Diagnosis and care of patients with anorexia nervosa in primary care settings. Ann Intern Med 134:1048–1059, 2001

Meyers DG, Starke H, Pearson PH, et al: Leaflet to left ventricular size disproportion and prolapse of a structurally normal mitral valve in anorexia nervosa. Am J Cardiol 60:911–914, 1987

Milosevic A: Eating disorders and the dentist. Br Dent J 186:109–113, 1999

Milosevic A, Brodie D, Slade PD: Dental erosion, oral hygiene, and nutrition in eating disorders. Int J Eat Disord 21:195–199, 1997

Mitchell JE, Boutacoff LI: Laxative abuse complicating bulimia: medical and treatment implications. Int J Eat Disord 5:325–334, 1986

Mitchell JE, Pyle RL, Eckert ED, et al: Electrolyte and other physiological abnormalities in patients with bulimia. Psychol Med 13:273–278, 1983

Mitchell JE, Pyle RL, Hatsukami K, et al: The dexamethasone suppression test in patients with bulimia. J Clin Psychiatry 45:508–511, 1984

Mitchell JE, Hatsukami D, Eckert ED, et al: Characteristics of 275 patients with bulimia. Am J Psychiatry 142:482–485, 1985

Mitchell JE, Seim HC, Colon E, et al: Medical complications and medical management of bulimia. Ann Intern Med 107:71–77, 1987a

Mitchell JE, Hatsukami D, Pyle RL, et al: Metabolic acidosis as a marker for laxative abuse in patients with bulimia. Int J Eat Disord 6:557–560, 1987b

Mitchell JE, Pomeroy C, Huber M: A clinician's guide to the eating disorders medicine cabinet. Int J Eat Disord 7:211–223, 1988a

Mitchell JE, Pomeroy C, Seppala M, et al: Pseudo-Bartter's syndrome, diuretic abuse, idiopathic edema and eating disorders. Int J Eat Disord 7:225–237, 1988b

Mitchell JE, Pyle RL, Hatsukami D, et al: Enema abuse as a clinical feature of bulimia nervosa. Psychosomatics 32:102–104, 1991

Morgan JF: Eating disorders and reproduction. Aust N Z Obstet Gynaecol 39:167–173, 1999

Morgan JF, Lacey JH, Sedgwick PM: Impact of pregnancy on bulimia nervosa. Br J Psychiatry 174:135–140, 1999

Mortola JF, Rasmussen DD, Yen SSC: Alterations of the adrenocorticotropin-cortisol axis in normal weight bulimic women: evidence for a central mechanism. J Clin Endocrinol Metab 68:517–522, 1989

Nagata T, Tobitani W, Kiriike N, et al: Capacity to produce cytokines during weight restoration in patients with anorexia nervosa. Psychosom Med 61:371–377, 1999

Nakao A, Isozaki H, Iwagaki H, et al: Gastric perforation caused by a bulimic attack in an anorexia nervosa patient: report of a case. Surg Today 30:435–437, 2000

National Institutes of Health: Clinical Guidelines on the Identification, Evaluation, and Treatment of Overweight and Obesity in Adults. Bethesda, MD, National Heart, Lung, and Blood Institute, 1998

National Institutes of Health Technology Assessment Conference Panel: Methods for voluntary weight loss and control. Ann Intern Med 116:942–949, 1992

Neumarker K-J: Mortality and sudden death in anorexia nervosa. Int J Eat Disord 21:205–212, 1997

Newman MM, Halmi KA: Relationship of bone density to estradiol and cortisol in anorexia nervosa and bulimia. Psychiatry Res 29:105–112, 1989

Palla B, Litt IF: Medical complications of eating disorders in adolescents. Pediatrics 81:613–623, 1988

Palmer EP, Guay AT: Reversible myopathy secondary to abuse of ipecac in patients with major eating disorders. N Engl J Med 313:1457–1459, 1985

Patton GC: Mortality in eating disorders. Psychol Med 18:947–951, 1988

Perlow JH, Morgan MA, Montgomery D, et al: Perinatal outcome in pregnancy complicated by massive obesity. Am J Obstet Gynecol 167:958–962, 1992

Pirke KM, Fichter MM, Chlond C, et al: Disturbances of the menstrual cycle in bulimia nervosa. Clin Endocrinol 27:245–251, 1987

Pi-Sunyer FX: The role of very-low-calorie diets in obesity. Am J Clin Nutr 56:240–243, 1992

Pomeroy C, Mitchell JE: Medical complications and management of eating disorders. Psychiatr Ann 19:488–493, 1989

Pomeroy C, Eckert E, Hu S, et al: Role of interleukin-6 and transforming growth factor-β in anorexia nervosa. Biol Psychiatry 36:836–839, 1994

Pomeroy C, Mitchell JE, Eckert E, et al: Effect of body weight and caloric restriction on serum complement proteins, including factor D/adipsin: studies in anorexia nervosa and obesity. Clin Exp Immunol 108:507–515, 1997

Rajala R, Partinen M, Sane T, et al: Obstructive sleep apnea syndrome in morbidly obese patients. J Intern Med 230:125–129, 1991

Ratnasuriya RH, Eisler I, Szmukler GI, et al: Anorexia nervosa: outcome and prognostic factors after 20 years. Br J Psychiatry 158:495–502, 1991

Rich LM, Caine MR, Findling JW, et al: Hypoglycemic coma in anorexia nervosa: case report and review of the literature. Arch Intern Med 150:894–95, 1990

Rigotti NA, Nussbaum SR, Herzog DB, et al: Osteoporosis in women with anorexia nervosa. N Engl J Med 311:1601–1606, 1984

Roberts MW, Li S-H: Oral findings in anorexia nervosa and bulimia nervosa: a study of 47 cases. J Am Dent Assoc 115:407–410, 1987

Robinson E, Bachrach LK, Katzman DK: Use of hormone replacement therapy to reduce the risk of osteopenia in adolescent girls with anorexia nervosa. J Adolesc Health 26:343–348, 2000

Rodin GM, Daneman D: Eating disorders and IDDM. Diabetes Care 15:1402–1412, 1992

Rossner S, Lagerstrand L, Persson HE: The sleep apnea syndrome in obesity: risk of sudden death. J Intern Med 230:135–141, 1991

Rubinstein I, Zamel N, DuBarry L, et al: Airflow limitation in morbidly obese, nonsmoking men. Ann Intern Med 112:828–832, 1991

Ryan CF, Whittaker JS, Road JD: Ventilatory dysfunction in severe anorexia nervosa. Chest 102:1286–1288, 1992

Rydall AC, Rodin GM, Olmsted MP, et al: Disordered eating behavior and microvascular complications in young women with insulin-dependent diabetes mellitus. N Engl J Med 336:1849–1854, 1997

Salisbury JJ, Mitchell JE: Bone mineral density and anorexia nervosa in women. Am J Psychiatry 148:768–774, 1991

Schocken DD, Holloway JD, Powers PS: Weight loss and the heart. Arch Intern Med 149:877–881, 1989

Seim HC, Mitchell JE, Pomeroy C, et al: Electrocardiographic findings associated with very low calorie dieting. Int J Obes Relat Metab Disord 19:817–819, 1995

Sharp CW, Freeman CPL: The medical complications of anorexia nervosa. Br J Psychiatry 162:452–462, 1993

Shiffman ML, Sugarman HJ, Kellum JM, et al: Gallstone formation after rapid weight loss: a prospective study in patients undergoing gastric bypass surgery for treatment of morbid obesity. Am J Gastroenterol 86:1000–1005, 1991

Simmons MS, Grayden SK, Mitchell JE: The need for psychiatric-dental liaison in the treatment of bulimia. Am J Psychiatry 143:783–784, 1986

Smith RRL, Spivak JL: Marrow cell necrosis in anorexia nervosa and involuntary starvation. Br J Haematol 60:525–530, 1985

Soyka LA, Grinspoon S, Levitsky LL, et al: The effects of anorexia nervosa on bone metabolism in female adolescents. J Clin Endocrinol Metab 84:4489–4496, 1999

Stewart DE: Reproductive functions in eating disorders. Ann Med 24:287–291, 1992

Strober M, Freeman R, Morrell W: The long-term course of severe anorexia nervosa in adolescents. Int J Eat Disord 22:339–360, 1997

Studen-Pavlovich D, Elliott MA: Eating disorders in women's oral health. Dent Clin North Am 45:491–511, 2001

Sugarman HJ, Fairman RP, Sood RK, et al: Long-term effects of gastric surgery for treating respiratory insufficiency of obesity. Am J Clin Nutr 55:597–601, 1992

Thomas MA, Rebar RW: The endocrinology of anorexia nervosa and bulimia nervosa. Curr Opin Obstet Gynecol 2:831–836, 1990

Turner J, Batik M, Palmer LJ, et al: Detection and importance of laxative abuse in adolescents with anorexia nervosa. J Am Acad Child Adolesc Psychiatry 39:375–385, 2000

Wada S, Nagase T, Koike Y, et al: A case of anorexia nervosa with acute renal failure induced by rhabdomyolysis; possible involvement of hypophosphatemia or phosphate depletion. Intern Med 31:478–482, 1992

Walsh JM, Wheat ME, Freund K: Detection, evaluation and treatment of eating disorders: the role of the primary care physician. J Gen Intern Med 15:577–590, 2000

Ward A, Troop N, Cachia M, et al: Doubly disabled: diabetes in combination with an eating disorder. Postgrad Med J 71:546–550, 1995

Ward A, Brown N, Treasure J: Persistent osteopenia after recovery from anorexia nervosa. Int J Eat Disord 22:71–75, 1997

Wilfley DE, Cohen LR: Psychological treatment of bulimia nervosa and binge eating disorder. Psychopharmacol Bull 33:437–454, 1997

Worobetz LJ, Inglis FG, Shaffer EA: The effect of ursodeoxycholic acid therapy on gallstone formation in the morbidly obese during rapid weight loss. Am J Gastroenterol 88:1705–1710, 1993

Zipfel S, Lowe B, Reas DL, et al: Long term prognosis in anorexia nervosa. Lancet 355:721–722, 2000

8

Alcohol and Drug Abuse

INTRODUCTION

A disturbingly high number of adults will develop alcohol abuse or dependence sometime during their lives, and many of these individuals will concomitantly abuse drugs. Others may abuse drugs but not alcohol. The rates of alcohol dependence and drug abuse are markedly higher in hospitalized medical and surgical patients and in patients with other psychiatric disorders (Allen et al. 1998). Thus the psychiatrist will frequently encounter patients with these problems in many practice settings (Cook et al. 1992; Galanter and Kleber 1994).

In this chapter we first focus on the role of the psychiatrist in the identification and management of medical problems secondary to alcohol abuse and dependence. We then turn to medical issues surrounding abuse and dependence on other drugs. We do not attempt to address diagnostic and screening techniques or pharmacotherapeutic strategies, as these are not germane to the purpose of this text and are covered extensively elsewhere.

The psychiatrist will often be the person best able to coordinate the medical care of patients who abuse drugs or alcohol. Doing so, it is hoped, will minimize the morbidity and mortality in both abstinent and nonabstinent patients. He or she will often work with a network of medical providers who are involved in various facets of the patient's medical management.

It should be remembered that one of the main reasons that addiction treatment developed outside mainstream medicine was the negative attitude of physicians toward alcoholic and drug-abusing patients. Many primary care physicians have regarded people struggling with addiction as having moral weakness and/or character deficits and, at times, as untreatable. Therefore, psychiatric providers often play an important role in coordinating care, serving as a source of education and motivation for the treatment team, and advocating for the patient.

ALCOHOL ABUSE AND DEPENDENCE

Excessive use of alcohol can result in a bewildering array of medical problems (MacDonald et al. 1996), negatively affecting nearly every organ system in the body. The severity of these negative effects can range from the mild to the life threatening. Likewise, the extent of alcohol consumption and length of time prior to the onset of these effects vary dramatically from individual to individual. Thus, the appropriate management of patients with alcohol use disorders requires not only familiarity with the literature about these disorders but also careful assessment of each individual as well as clinical experience and sound judgment (Severinghaus and Kinney 1996).

In this section we review the management of alcohol intoxication and withdrawal and the management of ongoing medical complications of alcohol misuse. However, before moving forward, we must first note that the most likely substance used by alcoholic individuals that can result in a fatal illness is not alcohol, but tobacco. Thus, it is incumbent on physicians involved in the care of these patients to address tobacco use as well. Patients in alcohol abuse treatment who receive concomitant smoking cessation treatment are more likely than those not receiving this intervention to stop smoking, and such treatment does not have a negative impact on the achievement of abstinence from alcohol (McIlvain et al. 1998). Alcoholic patients are far more likely to smoke than others in the general population (Dawson 2000; Zullino et al. 2000). Therefore, it is important that psychiatrists caring for patients with addictions develop and implement smoking-cessation strategies for these patients.

Assessment of Alcohol Intoxication

Some of the literature on the treatment of alcohol intoxication centers on the medical management of the patient brought to the emergency department in an alcohol-induced coma. Obviously, this situation will most likely be handled by the emergency department physician with little input from the psychiatrist (MacDonald et al. 1996). However, all psychiatrists are periodically confronted with an intoxicated patient who presents in the office or over the telephone. Because this scenario is more relevant to psychiatry and has been less extensively covered in traditional texts, we will focus on the evaluation of an intoxicated—but not stuporous or comatose—alcohol-using patient in the outpatient clinic or in a telephone-contact situation.

According to DSM-IV-TR (American Psychiatric Association 2000), to make the diagnosis of alcohol intoxication the clinician must document the recent ingestion of alcohol leading to behavioral changes such as impulsivity, labile mood, impaired judgment, and impaired social or occupational functioning (MacDonald et al. 1996). These dysfunctions must be accompanied by one of five signs of alcohol intoxication: slurred speech, impaired coordination, unsteady gait, nystagmus, or facial flushing.

During the evaluation process the clinician should focus on ascertaining certain pieces of information, including the following:

- amount of alcohol ingested
- rate of alcohol ingestion
- history of tolerance to the effects of alcohol
- history of signs or symptoms of dependence and serious withdrawal
- concomitant use of other drugs (therapeutic or nontherapeutic)
- potential for suicide, homicide, or an accident
- presence of other medical or psychiatric problems that could be exacerbated by the intoxication
- availability of a supportive but firm and caring person in the environment (e.g., social/familial environment) (Severinghaus and Kinney 1996).

Gathering this information is often difficult because the primary informant is intoxicated and therefore often uncooperative and, at times, unpredictable. Every effort should be made to access collateral sources of information.

The clinician should remember certain some basic facts about the pharmacokinetics of alcohol when evaluating a patient who has been drinking (Jones 2000; Li et al. 2000; Lieber and Abittin 1999; Mumenthaler et al. 1999). In an average 100-lb person, three "standard drinks" (one 12-oz can of beer, one 5-oz glass of wine, or one 1.5-oz shot of 80-proof liquor) are sufficient to achieve a blood alcohol level of 0.10%, whereas five such drinks are required in a 170-lb person. In general, women require less alcohol to reach this level, due to a higher percentage of body fat and lower levels of alcohol dehydrogenase in the gastric mucosa. However, the rate of drinking is also important. A typical 154-lb man who consumes one drink per hour is unlikely ever to achieve a blood alcohol level of 0.10%; if the same man had two drinks per hour, his blood alcohol level would progressively increase to potentially dangerous levels over time. It is also important to remember that the average person metabolizes alcohol at a rate of 0.025% per hour, a fact that allows the clinician to estimate the length of time until a subject will be in better control of motor and mental faculties.

The effects of a given level of alcohol in the blood vary widely depending on the tolerance of the user as well as the presence of other drugs and medical conditions. In general, by considering the severity of the effects of the ingested alcohol on behavior (i.e., evaluating changes in mood, speech, coordination) as well as information on the rate and amount of alcohol ingestion, a clinician can make a reasonable estimate as to the level of alcohol in the blood. However, psychiatrists who work in clinical situations where accurate and exact determination of levels is necessary should have a Breathalyzer available and staff trained to use it appropriately.

It is also helpful to be able to correlate behavioral effects with a given blood alcohol level (Severinghaus and Kinney 1996). If a patient presents with minimal behavioral symptoms yet has a highly elevated blood alcohol level, one can deduce a high degree of tolerance and probably significant alcohol dependence.

It is also important in the evaluation process to determine whether the patient fulfills criteria for alcohol dependence. The more severely dependent patient will be less likely to stop drinking, despite remonstrations to the contrary. Also, those with a history of severe withdrawal symptoms will require more highly structured and medically skilled settings for detoxification. However, the less dependent patient with a high blood alcohol level is actually at greater risk of dying secondary to respiratory depression.

It is critical that the use of other drugs (therapeutic or nontherapeutic) also be evaluated, because use of alcohol not only correlates with increased usage of other recreational drugs but also can result in negative interactions with a wide variety of prescribed drugs (Severinghaus and Kinney 1996). Most critical in intoxication is alcohol's potentiation of the sedative and respiratory-depressant effects of central nervous system (CNS)–depressant drugs. Because of this, blood alcohol levels not usually associated with severe CNS depression can lead to stupor or coma when alcohol is used with other CNS depressants. If unacknowledged use of other drugs is suspected, a toxicology screen should be conducted. Other important drug interactions include exacerbation of the hepatotoxicity in acetaminophen overdose, and the potential for aged beers and wines to cause a tyramine reaction when used with monoamine oxidase inhibitors.

Another critical assessment to be made with the intoxicated patient is the risk of injury to self or others. Intoxicated individuals are much more likely to engage in violent acts against self or others. A high percentage of motor vehicle accidents, incidents of domestic violence, and completed suicides occur in the context of alcohol intoxication, and 10% of patients with alcohol dependence will eventually die by suicide. Unfortunately, these events are difficult to predict. Thus, threats of violent acts by an intoxicated patient must be taken seriously. Also, the clinician must assess intoxicated subjects for traumatic injuries due to fights or accidents.

In evaluating suicide potential, psychiatric symptomatology should also be assessed. Simply put, intoxication, as well as chronic use of alcohol, exacerbates the course of non-substance-induced mental disorders. Intoxication and chronic use of alcohol not only affect important neural substrates involved in the mechanisms of psychiatric disorders but also result in decreased compliance with psychiatric treatments. A simple rule of thumb is that a psychiatric disorder should be considered more severe in the presence of substance intoxication, abuse, or dependence. The assessment and management of the intoxicated patient is made much easier by the presence of a reliable, nonintoxicated relative or friend. Unfortunately, such patients are often alienated from others in their environment, and at times those from whom information is sought are also intoxicated. Therefore, the clinician must assess the reliability of the history obtained from others.

A difficult but all-too-frequent situation occurs when the clinician is dealing with an intoxicated patient by phone and concludes that an in-person evaluation is necessary. Transportation by a nonintoxicated driver should be arranged, even if this requires calling an ambulance or arranging police intervention. This may require the use of emergency legal holds or promises (not threats) to call police and report that the patient is driving under the influence of alcohol.

Management of Alcohol Intoxication

Decisions must be made about the appropriate setting and the proper approach for the treatment of alcohol intoxication (Severinghaus and Kinney 1996). Most frequently, hospital admission is justified if there is a possible need for resuscitation and other medical support in individuals with alcohol-induced coma, if the behavioral disturbances induced by alcohol render the patient a danger to self or others, or if concerns exist about a severe withdrawal syndrome that would require inpatient management.

Most often, psychiatrists are involved in assessing alcohol-induced behavioral syndromes, which can involve mood lability, impaired judgment, violence, lack of coordination, confusion, hallucinations, and paranoia. This is best dealt with by providing a safe place in which the patient can stay until the alcohol level declines.

The onset of delusions (referred to as alcohol-induced psychotic disorder in DSM-IV-TR) or hallucinations (usually auditory, but possibly visual in a syndrome known as alcoholic hallucinosis) can begin during a drinking bout or during withdrawal. These symptoms, usually occuring in the presence of a clear sensorium, generally resolve within a few days to a few weeks. The symptoms may be of sufficient severity to dictate the use of neuroleptic therapy (e.g., haloperidol in doses as high as 20 mg/day, although lower doses will usually suffice). The clinician should remember that antipsychotics will decrease seizure threshold. Treatment of hallucinosis almost invariably requires a hospital setting as these patients are not likely to be cooperative with outpatient detoxification.

Assessment of Alcohol Withdrawal

Alcohol withdrawal is a potentially life-threatening syndrome that usually occurs when a chronic heavy drinker significantly decreases or ceases alcohol intake abruptly. It is particularly likely to occur when drinking suddenly ceases after an episode of binge drinking. However, given the seriousness of withdrawal, and the difficulty in obtaining reliable information about duration of drinking in heavy drinkers, it is best to be conservative and assume that even shorter drinking bouts may be sufficient to result in serious withdrawal symptoms.

Alcohol withdrawal often occurs when a heavy drinker or alcohol-dependent person becomes physically ill or incapacitated and stops drinking suddenly. Withdrawal from alcohol can occur in patients admitted to medical/surgical service when the severity of drinking has not been appreciated. Moreover, in such medical and surgical settings, the onset of the symptoms of alcohol withdrawal is often confused with changes in the primary illness for which the patient was admitted. Therefore, such withdrawal may progress to more dangerous levels before it is diagnosed. One way that psychiatrists can prevent this occurrence is to advocate for the universal use of screening instruments for alcohol dependence, such as the CAGE interview, in their practice organizations.

Management of Alcohol Withdrawal

To effectively treat alcohol withdrawal, providers must have a high level of suspicion regarding the possibility of this diagnosis. Providers must also understand the time course and pathophysiology of withdrawal, its signs and symptoms, and the proper setting as well as pharmacologic strategies for its management. The goal of the treatment of alcohol withdrawal is to either prevent the episode or minimize the severity of symptoms.

There are four major syndromes for which patients must be monitored during early abstinence: withdrawal (minor and major), seizures, alcohol hallucinosis, and Wernicke's encephalopathy. Because all of these syndromes occur in roughly the same time period, the interventions described for each syndrome must usually be prescribed simultaneously (Gallant 1994). It is also critical to remember that alcohol withdrawal is often associated with other systemic illnesses (e.g., alcohol-related pancreatitis, gastrointestinal bleeding, and hepatitis).

The earliest symptoms of alcohol withdrawal (also referred to as minor symptoms) include a coarse tremor of the hands, tongue, or eyelids (the most frequently noticed early sign of withdrawal), gastrointestinal symptoms, and changes in mood and sleep. Alcohol withdrawal can progress to a more lethal syndrome known as delirium tremens (DTs), in which disorientation, confusion, and disordered perception are combined with autonomic dysregulation marked by tachycardia, profuse sweating, and flushing. These symptoms usually peak 2–3 days after abstinence begins and resolve after 3–5 days.

Other symptoms can emerge early in the abstinence phase. Seizures or "rum fits" occur as early as 6 hours after the last drink and almost always occur within the first 48 hours (MacDonald et al. 1996). The occurrence of seizures indicates an increased risk of subsequent DTs, but even if a seizure occurs, most patients do not go on to develop DTs. Less than 5% of withdrawal seizures progress to status epilepticus. Importantly, seizures can be the first sign of withdrawal, and a history of withdrawal seizures should result in more aggressive treatment methods.

Alcoholic hallucinosis can also begin during the withdrawal phase and can be differentiated from DTs by the presence of a clear sensorium (MacDonald et al. 1996). Wernicke's encephalopathy is characterized by confusion (like DTs), but the confusion is accompanied by ophthalmoplegia (lateral rectus palsies and conjugate gaze palsies) and ataxia (Smith 1986b). Finally, Wernicke's encephalopathy (usually followed by Korsakoff's syndrome or alcohol amnestic disorder) also has its onset during the first few days after abstinence begins.

After the identification of a patient at risk for withdrawal, the first decision that must be made is whether the patient meets criteria for hospitalization for detoxification. These criteria include the following:

- severe tremulousness
- hallucinosis
- fever over 101°F
- seizures (in a patient without a history of seizure disorder)
- evidence of delirium or Wernicke's encephalopathy
- any significant head trauma
- presence of a significant comorbid acute medical or psychiatric syndrome
- history of severe withdrawal with seizures, delirium, or psychosis
- lack of availability of a sober, cooperative support person

However, the reason most frequently cited as an indication for inpatient detoxification is the lack of a supportive, structured environment. This problem can be overcome by creating alternative sites that can support individuals experiencing uncomplicated detoxification, such as "lodger" units within hospital campuses.

To appropriately manage patients, pretreatment evaluation requires laboratory examination including a toxicology screen; complete blood count with differential; serum magnesium, phosphorus, electrolytes, and glucose; hepatic and renal functions; and protime. Patients at risk for alcohol withdrawal can be dehydrated, hypokalemic, hyponatremic, or hypoglycemic. Depending on the extent of these problems, the patient may require intravenous fluid and electrolyte replacement.

A baseline score on the Clinical Institute Withdrawal Assessment for Alcohol, Revised (CIWA-Ar, MacDonald et al. 1996) should be obtained. On this scale patients are scored on 10 different attributes of alcohol withdrawal. The regular use of the CIWA-Ar leads to improved consistency in the treatment of alcohol withdrawal symptoms by all staff members. It also provides a broader assessment of the multiple types of signs and symptoms possible in withdrawal and helps avoid undertreatment of patients with atypical presentations. An alternative instrument is the Alcohol Withdrawal Scale (AWS).

The following recommendations are based on work by MacDonald et al. (1996). Individuals who have CIWA-Ar scores of less than 6 may be adequately treated with supportive care alone but require regular reassessment (e.g., every 8 hours for 24 hours). Patients who score between 6 and 11 are typically given the equivalent of 10 mg of diazepam and are reassessed in no more than 8 hours. Individuals with scores higher than 11 require the equivalent of 10 mg of diazepam but must be reassessed every 1–2 hours. The goal of benzodiazepine treatment is to provide a partial replacement for alcohol's γ-aminobuytric acid–mediated CNS depressant effects and a mild level of sedation during the most severe parts of withdrawal, and to avoid progression to more severe variants of withdrawal. Benzodiazepines with longer half-lives such as diazepam or chlordiazepoxide are well suited to this goal because their use allows the clinician to avoid fluctuations between excessive and insufficient sedation that can trigger drug-seeking behavior on the part of the patient. In addition, long-half-life drugs will be gradually cleared and still provide some antiwithdrawal protection in the event that an impulsive patient decides to leave the hospital prematurely. Short- and intermediate-half-life benzodiazepines such as lorazepam are more appropriate than long-half-life benzodiazepines in some patients. Intravenous benzodiazepines can be used if patients cannot or will not take medications by mouth. The most common indication for their use is in patients with compromised liver function (usually from cirrhosis) or the need for intramuscular treatment due to profound nausea. Although these medications can be used in outpatient detoxification, it is necessary to have a competent adult available to prevent the patient from having to drive or engage in any activity that is dangerous to perform when sedated.

Relatively recently, studies have also confirmed that carbamazepine is effective not only for seizure prophylaxis but also for treatment of autonomic arousal caused by alcohol withdrawal (Erstad and Cotugno 1995; Gallant 1994; Ozdemir et al. 1994). Carbamazepine can be started at 200 mg four times a day in most patients and given for 48 hours with a subsequent taper over 6 days. This drug must be used cautiously in those with hepatic dysfunction. Alternate strategies for managing withdrawal employ barbiturates or beta-blockers. However, barbiturates have tended to be used infrequently due to their lower therapeutic index and the fact that modern clinicians are less familiar with this class of drugs. Beta-blockers, such as atenolol (50–100 mg), have been shown to decrease the peripheral autonomic effects (e.g., tachycardia) of withdrawal, but these drugs do not provide protection against the progression to DTs and should not be used as the sole pharmacologic intervention in detoxification (MacDonald et al. 1996).

Seizures tend to occur early in the course of the withdrawal, often in the first 24 hours and after as few as 6 hours (MacDonald et al. 1996). If a patient has a history of seizures, antiseizure treatment should be started preemptively. Both benzodiazepines and carbamazepine are effective anticonvulsants in this context; phenytoin, however, does not have established efficacy in this regard (Gallant 1994). A typical strategy for benzodiazepine seizure prophylaxis would be diazepam 10 mg every 6 hours for 24 hours with subsequent taper beginning 48 hours after the last drink. The onset of seizures should also reinvigorate the search for metabolic problems, especially electrolyte and magnesium abnormalities, and any such abnormalities should be corrected promptly via intravenous replacement. The occurrence of a single withdrawal seizure does not necessitate anticonvulsant therapy long term.

Despite adequate intervention, some patients may progress to DTs. This may also occur when patients present late in their course of withdrawal (Gallant 1994). DTs can be thought of as an autonomic "storm," with associated psychotic delirium. This potentially life-threatening condition requires management by physicians and a health care team familiar with this syndrome. The onset of delirium, especially if accompanied by a fever of more than 101°F, should prompt further examination to uncover any underlying medical problems. An intravenous line should be started, and fluids should be given as needed to replace losses from sweating as well as gastrointestinal losses. Physical restraints should be readily available. The usual treatment approach is use of intravenous lorazepam 2 mg and haloperidol 5 mg, with dosing as frequently as every 30 minutes, the aim being to keep the patient sedated for about 3 days. The use of this aggressive sedation strategy requires attention to possible respiratory depression and other consequences of oversedation.

Administering parenteral , and then later oral, thiamine 100 mg/day is critical in the prevention and/or treatment of Wernicke's encephalopathy and the frequently co-occurring Korsakoff's psychosis (or alcoholic amnestic disorder). One must be careful to administer thiamine prior to the administration of glucose solutions because glucose administration to a thiamine-deficient patient may acutely precipitate the onset of Wernicke's syndrome.

Management of Other Medical Problems

Outpatient management by the clinician of medical problems related to drug and alcohol abuse, categorized by organ system, is discussed below. Findings on the review of systems during history taking or laboratory tests may suggest alcohol abuse and trigger further diagnostic procedures. Suggestions for laboratory testing are presented in Table 8–1, including possible interpretation and diagnostic and treatment steps.

Gastrointestinal

Alcohol exerts harmful effects on the gastrointestinal system at various levels (Fenster 1986; Worthington-Roberts 1986).

Esophagus and Stomach. Heavy alcohol use decreases gastric peristalsis and lowers the sphincter pressure at the gastroesophageal junction (Fenster 1986). This increases the chance of leakage of acidic gastric con-

Table 8–1. Laboratory parameters in alcoholic patients

Parameters	When and why to order	Abnormality	Diagnostic interpretation	Response
Serum glutamic-oxaloacetic transaminase (SGOT; 1–36 u/L) Gamma-glutamyltransferase (GGT; 5–40 u/L) Serum glutamate pyruvate transaminase (SGPT; 1–45 u/L)	Baseline and tracking	Elevated	Ethanol abuse, rule out alcoholic hepatitis and cirrhosis	Gastrointestinal consultation
Serum amylase (25–125 u/L)	Abdominal or back pain	Elevated	Pancreatitis	Pain relief, gastrointestinal consultation, nothing by mouth, nasogastric suction
Serum magnesium (1.3–2.1 mg/dL)	Withdrawal	Reduced	Hypomagnesemia	Replace
Complete blood count with differential (hemoglobin-M, 13–18 g/dL; hemoglobin-F, 12–16 g/dL)	Baseline; also if hematemesis, melena	Reduced hemoglobin and hematocrit	Anemia, rule out bleeding and malnutrition	Consider internal medicine consultation, depends on etiology
Guaic (neg)	Baseline; also if hematemesis, melena	Positive	Gastrointestinal bleeding	Gastrointestinal consultation
Serum ammonia (NH_3; 10–50 mmol/L)	Memory problems, confusion, cirrhosis	Elevated	Hepatic encephalopathy	Gastrointestinal consultation, restrict protein, consider neomycin or metronidazole
Folic acid B_{12} (145–540 ng/mL, 180–900 pg/mL)	Neuropathy, anemia (especially elevated mean corpuscular volume), memory problems	Reduced	Deficiency	Replace

tents (e.g., reflux) into the esophagus, which can result in heartburn pain and, potentially, Barrett's esophagus (MacDonald et al. 1996). Heavy alcohol use can also lead to irritation of the stomach because alcohol disrupts the protective gastric mucosal barrier, which can lead to hematemesis or melena but more frequently is simply evidenced by epigastric pain, often relieved by antacids. Peptic ulcer, pancreatitis, hepatitis, and other abdominal disorders must be ruled out. There is little evidence that alcohol causes classic gastric or duodenal ulcers. However, if gastritis is sufficiently severe, it can progress to ulceration. Severe gastritis can result in retching and vomiting of sufficient severity to cause Mallory-Weiss syndrome, in which the gastrointestinal mucosa ruptures at or near the gastroesophageal junction. This condition sometimes requires surgery but is often self-limited. Rarely, retching can lead to a frank rupture of the lower esophagus (Boerhaave's syndrome), an intensely painful surgical emergency and often fatal.

The rate of esophageal cancer is markedly elevated in heavy drinkers who also smoke (MacDonald et al. 1996). The diagnosis is usually made by esophagram or endoscopy after symptoms of dysphagia or weight loss prompt investigation.

Liver. It is important to note that there is wide variation in the severity and clinical significance of liver changes induced by heavy drinking (Crabb 1999; Lieber 2000). Many patients with evidence of liver damage may not go on to develop cirrhosis and liver failure. However, cirrhosis continues to be one of the top 10 causes of death in the United States.

About a quarter of heavy drinkers develop an elevation in gamma-glutamyltransferase (GGT), and, conversely, about 70% of patients with elevated GGT abuse alcohol. GGT levels correct after 3–6 months of abstinence; persistent elevation should occasion a search for alternate causes. In some asymptomatic patients there is also an accumulation of fat in the liver known as alcoholic fatty liver or steatosis. Most often this condition resolves with abstinence as well.

In some heavy alcohol users, liver abnormalities progress beyond fatty infiltration to cell death and inflammation consistent with hepatitis (Lieber 1998). The onset can be acute or gradual and associated with signs of liver inflammation and dysfunction. Symptoms include right upper quadrant pain, nausea, and malaise; signs include a tender, enlarged liver, jaundice, and fever; and laboratory tests include elevated liver function tests (with aspartate aminotrasferase > alanine aminotransferase) and hyperbilirubinemia (Lieber 1998). The acute symptoms and signs often resolve with abstinence, but it is probable that the liver incurs permanent scarring with each episode of inflammation and that repeated episodes can lead to cirrhosis and liver failure (Worthington-Roberts 1986).

The end stage of the inflammatory/scarring process is alcoholic cirrhosis (Lieber 2000). In this condition liver tissue is replaced by fibroses, with resultant nodule formation that can obliterate the normal lobular liver structure. Cirrhosis may be confirmed by liver biopsy. The key symptoms and signs that develop over and above those of intermittent alcoholic hepatitis are those related to portal hypertension and shunting of blood around the liver. This results in a failure to detoxify blood-borne metabolites, resulting in hepatic encephalopathy and enlargement of esophageal, hemorrhoidal, and periumbilical veins that are alternate routes of blood around the liver. The dilated esophageal veins or esophageal varices can bleed, causing hematemesis that can be life threatening. Portal hypertension can also lead to splenic enlargement and consequent sequestration of white blood cells, resulting in neutropenia.

Elevated serum ammonia levels are not sufficient to confirm the diagnosis of hepatic encephalopathy, but changes in serum ammonia level can be correlated with symptom severity in some patients. Treatment of hepatic encephalopathy includes dietary protein restriction and decreasing gastrointestinal sources of ammonia by use of neomycin or metronidazole and lactulose.

Liver damage due to cirrhosis also results in a decrease in synthesis of albumin and prothrombin. These changes lead to the signs and symptoms of ascites (actually a consequence of the interaction of hypoalbuminemia and portal hypertension), resulting in loss of fluid from intravascular space and bruising (probably related to alcohol-induced decreases in platelets). Ascites is usually treated by dietary sodium restriction (to 2–4 g/day), fluid restriction (to about 1.5 L/day), and careful diuretic treatment. About 20% of patients with cirrhosis due to alcohol will develop a hepatoma (primary liver cancer).

Psychiatrists who are involved in the treatment of alcoholic patients and who work in major medical centers are sometimes consulted regarding the appropriateness of liver transplant (Beresford 1997; Keeffe 1996; Lucey 1993). Transplant outcomes in patients with liver failure due to alcohol have consistently been as good as or better than those achieved in patients with liver failure from other causes. The psychiatrist practicing in this arena should become familiar with current standards for pretransplant sobriety and involvement in pro-abstinence activities.

Pancreas. Alcohol-induced pancreatic problems include both acute and chronic pancreatitis (Fenster 1986; Isla 2000; Munoz and Katerndahl 2000; Pitchumoni 1998). The precise mechanism by which alcohol induces pancreatitis is unclear. Symptoms include upper abdominal pain, nausea and vomiting, ileus, and occasionally hypovolemia. Elevated serum amylase and/or lipase in a patient with these symptoms allows a presumptive diagnosis of acute pancreatitis. Manifestations may include peripheral fat necrosis, obstructive jaundice, pseudocyst development, or acute hypovolemia (Amurawaiye and Brown 1991). Treatment for acute pancreatitis generally consists of putting the bowel at rest by stopping oral intake and using nasogastric suction plus analgesia. Meperidine is the preferred narcotic for analgesia because it does not cause spasm of the sphincter of Oddi.

Chronic pancreatitis is characterized by chronic pain, bouts of acute pain, and/or endocrine and exocrine insufficiencies such as hypoinsulinemia resulting in diabetes mellitus and insufficient production of digestive enzymes resulting in malabsorption. The management of chronic and frequently recurrent pain in patients with a history of addiction to alcohol (and often other drugs) is a problem for treatment providers (Portenoy and Payne 1997). Clearly, nonnarcotic analgesics should be tried. If these fail, narcotics can be considered if a clear contract about the amount of narcotics, the time periods of prescriptions, and the rules about changing prescriptions and handling crises can be negotiated. Endocrine and exocrine insufficiencies are handled by replacement of enzymes and hormones. Pancreatic enzyme supplements generally contain lipase, amylase, and proteases and are taken before each meal. Insulin replacement using established diabetic guidelines may be needed. It is vital that the clinician involved in the care of alcoholic patients determine whether the patient with chronic pancreatitis can follow this complicated replacement regimen, and arrange greater environmental support and structure if the alcoholic patient cannot manage independently.

Small and Large Intestine. The deleterious effect of alcohol on the mucosa of the small intestine can cause malabsorption and diarrhea (Lieber 1998) as well as symptoms of irritable bowel syndrome (Masand et al. 1998). The stools resulting from dysfunction of the small intestine are frequent and loose, not large, not malodorous, and not fatty as are those resulting from pancreatic insufficiency. This state of malabsorption and chronic diarrhea can result in electrolyte and magnesium deficiencies, rectal fissures and perianal itching, and folate and other vitamin deficiencies. Treatment requires abstinence from alcohol, replacement of deficiencies in vitamins and electrolytes, and, occasionally, use of antidiarrheals to slow frequency of loose stools. Hemorrhoids due to portal hypertension can be another source of rectal discomfort and bleeding. Usual topical treatments are used, but surgical intervention is at times required.

Cardiovascular

Alcohol abuse appears to significantly increase the risk of hypertension. Alcohol also appears to have direct toxic effects on cardiac as well as skeletal muscle (Maisch 1996; Rubin and Urbano-Marquez 1994; Schenker and Bay 1998; Smith 1986a). Symptoms such as dyspnea, orthopnea, and decreased exercise tolerance and signs such as edema, a third heart sound, and jugular venous distension are all consistent with alcoholic cardiomyopathy (MacDonald et al. 1996). Chest X-ray findings of congestive heart failure and an enlarged heart and echocardiogram studies consistent with a decrease of ventricle wall thickness and motion are consistent with alcoholic cardiomyopathy. Absolute abstinence from alcohol plus treatment with standard congestive heart failure interventions are indicated.

As many as one-fifth of patients with atrial arrhythmias are thought to have the problem secondary to chronic alcohol use. Recurrent atrial arrhythmias should raise the issue of possible alcohol abuse.

Neurologic

Central Nervous System. Excessive alcohol use is associated with a variety of types of insults to the brain including the following:

- trauma due to altercations while intoxicated
- trauma due to accidents resulting from problems with coordination and gait
- atrophy of neurons
- hepatic encephalopathy due to nitrogenous toxins
- hypoglycemia
- thiamine deficiency (Kushner 1991)

The clinician does not usually see a pure case of the disorders described below but rather a mixture of signs and symptoms reflecting a variety of negative effects of alcohol on the brain.

Trauma can result not only in the sequelae of closed head injuries but also in subdural hematomas. Signs and symptoms of frontal lobe dysfunction such as apathy, personality change, and disorders of executive function as well as signs of increased intracranial pressure are often observed. Neurosurgical consultation including computed tomography (CT) or magnetic resonance imaging (MRI) confirmation as well as surgical drainage is required.

Dementia due to alcohol use is thought to reflect diffuse neuronal death due to both direct and indirect effects of alcohol (Lieber 1998;

Oslin et al. 1998). Because initial changes can be subtle, it is wise to use a standardized screening instrument such as the Mini-Mental Status Examination when evaluating heavy drinkers. These examinations should be repeated after a few days or weeks of abstinence to establish a baseline not distorted by the effects of intoxication or withdrawal. Atrophy can be seen by CT or MRI scanning. This disorder is usually of insidious onset and therefore difficult to distinguish from Alzheimer's disease. Again, abstinence from alcohol is vital, and thiamine supplementation should be started immediately to reverse or prevent progression of any component attributable to Wernicke-Korsakoff syndrome.

Wernicke's encephalopathy is characterized by ataxia, confusion and excitation, and paralysis of extraocular muscles (Smith 1986b). It is caused by a relative thiamine deficiency that leads to petechial lesions affecting the mammillary bodies as well as other parts of the brain. Confusion and excitation are the most frequent early symptoms and often occur in alcoholic patients who have evidence of peripheral neuropathy. Abnormal extraocular movement differentiates this alcohol-induced confusional state from intoxication and withdrawal. Thiamine administration is critical for the reversal of this syndrome; hypomagnesemia should also be addressed. It is vital that thiamine be given to the alcoholic patient prior to the start of any glucose infusion as the increase in carbohydrate metabolism increases the body's demand for thiamine and can precipitate Wernicke's encephalopathy.

Unfortunately, Wernicke's encephalopathy is often followed by the onset of Korsakoff's psychosis (or alcohol amnestic syndrome) (Smith 1986b). Korsakoff's—misnamed because the problem is one of amnesia, not psychosis—is characterized by an anterograde amnesia with confabulation. Thiamine replacement (50–100 mg/day) is vital.

Cerebellar degeneration tends to occur in severe, chronic alcoholic patients with poor nutrition. Physical examination will reveal a broad-based gait, impaired heel-shin testing, and often a mild tremor. CT or MRI scans can be used to document cerebellar atrophy. Abstinence and good nutrition optimize the chance for at least some improvement.

Peripheral Nervous System. Peripheral neuropathy may be caused by insufficient B vitamin intake (D'Amour and Butterworth 1994; Diamond and Messing 1994). This disorder is characterized by a bilateral stocking-and-glove distribution of sensory dysfunction. Deficits in deep tendon reflexes, two-point or vibratory discrimination, and proprioception are found on physical examination. Complaints of burning pain, tingling, or numbness occur early, and later these sensory complaints are accompanied by muscle wasting (Smith 1986b). Electromyogram and nerve conduction studies can confirm the neuropathy, but other causes of neuropathy must be ruled out. Again, abstinence and good nutrition plus vitamin supplements are indicated.

Hematologic and Immunologic

Alcohol use negatively affects the production as well as the survival of various blood cell lines. The most frequent hematologic issues encountered are anemia, thrombocytopenia, and neutropenia (Hillman 1986).

Anemia must be carefully evaluated in alcoholic patients because they have multiple potential sites for blood loss (e.g., varices, gastritis) as well as multiple types of nutritional deficits (iron, B_{12}, folate) (Fernando and Grimsley 1998). Microcytic anemias are often due to iron deficiency and can reflect poor intake or slow blood loss. The clinician is obligated to rule out all potential sites of bleeding prior to simply replacing iron. Normocytic anemia is often secondary to alcohol's toxic effects on erythropoiesis, or bleeding. Macrocytic anemias are most likely due to folic acid or B_{12} deficiencies, although alcohol can induce a macrocytic anemia without these deficiencies.

Thrombocytopenia, with platelet counts as low as 30,000–50,000, can occur, reflecting both bone marrow suppression by alcohol and sequestration of platelets in the spleen. Abstinence usually reverses this. Acute replacement is usually needed only when there are clear signs of bleeding.

Alcohol, as well as folic acid deficiency, can adversely affect the production and function of neutrophils. This might explain the vulnerability of alcoholic patients to overwhelming pneumococcal sepsis.

Endocrinologic

Alcoholic males and females demonstrate signs and symptoms of primary gonadal atrophy. In males, testes are often smaller and softer than normal. Blood estrogen is sometimes elevated, leading to gynecomastia, loss of body hair, and spider angiomas. Impotence is much more frequent than in nonalcoholic populations. Alcoholic women experience decreased fertility and early menopause.

Dermatologic

Jaundice reflects the hyperbilirubinemia of liver failure. Petechiae suggest alcohol-induced thrombocytopenia, whereas palmar erythema provides a clue to chronic alcohol use in a patient who is denying the behavior. Cigarette burns on the fingers are suggestive not only of severe intoxication but also neuropathy.

DRUG ABUSE AND DEPENDENCE

This section focuses on the medical issues clinicians should consider in working with patients who abuse drugs (Novick et al. 1997). It is not intended to provide a definitive account of diagnostic or treatment strategies for all the possible medical conditions that can develop, but instead is intended to provide a useful set of principles in treating these patients.

Alcohol and nicotine are the two most widely used drugs in the United States. They are clearly those associated with the greatest medical morbidity and mortality; chronic use of either one often results in illness. The drugs discussed in this chapter, however, are most likely to be associated with medical problems during intoxication and withdrawal. The intravenous route of administration in cocaine, heroin, or amphetamine use carries its own risks. We review the intoxication and withdrawal effects, as well as the medical problems of intravenous drug use, as they relate to use of cocaine and other stimulants, heroin, hallucinogens, and phencyclidine (PCP).

Two caveats are important at the outset. First, although we discuss the medical problems associated with each drug individually, one should always assume that multiple substances are involved, as polysubstance abuse is the rule, not the exception. Second, abuse of drugs as well as alcohol can mimic nearly all forms of psychopathology. Therefore, the clinician must strongly consider substance abuse in the differential diagnosis of virtually every patient evaluated. Furthermore, toxicity screens can be very useful in identifying drug-abusing patients. The use of these screening tests is described more fully below.

Cocaine and Other Stimulants

Although the abuse of both cocaine and amphetamines can be characterized by a chronic, low-dose, daily pattern of use, it often escalates to a pattern in which the drug is smoked or used intravenously in high dosages during binges (Kerfoot et al. 1996). These binges last from a few hours to a few days and usually end when the patient runs out of drugs and money or collapses.

Intoxication is marked by increased feelings of well-being or frank euphoria, increased energy, and signs of autonomic arousal (Kerfoot et al. 1996). Other effects include decreased sleep, decreased appetite, and increased sexual drive. Sometimes patients report dramatic improvements in concentration, and some will report a calming effect. In such cases, a thorough history regarding attention deficit disorder is recommended. Chronic use of stimulants can lead to paranoia, anxiety, or panic as opposed to the euphoria of early use (Kushner 1991). Such states can be difficult to differentiate from other disorders such as panic disorder and schizophrenia.

The physical signs of intoxication include tachycardia, hypertension, increased respiratory rate, and increased body temperature. If the patient is vulnerable, or if the level of ingestion is high, seizures and cardiovascular collapse can occur (Kushner 1991). Myocardial infarction or arrhythmia can lead to death or ongoing morbidity (Boghdadi and Henning 1997; Kerfoot et al. 1996).

Many difficulties can arise in the assessment of cardiac status in patients who abuse stimulants. First, intoxicated patients often do not pay much attention to chest discomfort and may have a "silent" myocardial infarction. Electrocardiograms on patients with a history of cocaine ingestion at times reveal evidence of past myocardial ischemia. Second, chest pain often arises while the patient is experiencing panic-like symptoms, and this may lead the clinician to overlook its importance.

Other physical signs and symptoms found in stimulant abusers are those attributable to cerebrovascular accidents or transient ischemic attacks (Kerfoot et al. 1996; Petitti et al. 1998). Again, imaging of the brains of stimulant abusers can show evidence of "silent" ischemic events, probably related to stimulant-induced hypertension or vasospasm. A thorough mental status and neurologic examination is important if a central ischemic event is suspected. Other important acute medical problems seen in stimulant intoxication include dyspnea due to spontaneous pneumothorax or crack hypersensitivity and traumatic injuries not apparent to the intoxicated patient.

A critical physical sign to evaluate is weight loss. As cocaine and amphetamines decrease appetite, weight loss is often accepted as a logical consequence of drug use. However, given the prevalence of HIV and other infections related to unsafe sexual practices and intravenous drug use, weight loss should always be considered a possible sign of infection (see Chapter 2). Finally, because cocaine is sometimes used by patients with eating disorders to control appetite, weight loss or abnormal eating behaviors should trigger questioning regarding a possible eating disorder (see Chapter 7).

The existence of a withdrawal syndrome related to cocaine has been hotly debated for years (Kerfoot et al. 1996). Although the early states of abstinence from cocaine can clearly be uncomfortable for some patients, withdrawal from cocaine is clearly not lethal, and newly abstinent patients often report very few symptoms.

Gawin and colleagues (Gawin 1991; Gawin and Khalsa-Denison 1996; O'Malley and Gawin 1990) have described a three-stage process of withdrawal from cocaine. The first stage, termed the "crash" phase, is characterized by mild to severe depression, anxiety, anhedonia, changes in sleep, increased appetite, and slowed psychomotor function. Some patients continue to display cocaine-induced psychotic symptoms, and some are sufficiently agitated to require treatment. Sometimes antipsychotics are necessary, but the use of these should be limited while cocaine is still in the patient's system because both drugs decrease seizure threshold. The first stage lasts a few hours to 4 days, blending into the second stage, which is termed *withdrawal.* During this period, which lasts for roughly 10 weeks, sleep patterns improve, but the patient experiences fatigue, anxiety, and decreased ability to enjoy activities. Drug craving during this time can lead to treatment cessation and relapse. The third stage is characterized by an improvement in mood and decrease in anhedonia, but cravings can persist. Most pharmacotherapeutic efforts have been designed for use during the second or third stage.

There are no significant medical problems related directly to cocaine withdrawal. However, cocaine is frequently used in conjunction with alcohol. While many use alcohol to moderate anxiety or agitation due to cocaine ingestion, the body can metabolize simultaneously ingested cocaine and alcohol to a substance (cocaethylene) capable of creating a cocaine-like high, but with a longer half-life. This suggests that some patients use the combination in pursuit of a better high. However, abstinence from both substances puts the patient at risk for not only the discomfort of cocaine withdrawal but also mortality from alcohol withdrawal.

Opiates

Intoxication with heroin and/or other opiates results in a brief period of euphoria followed by sedation (Hirsh et al. 1996). The rate of onset and decline of these effects varies as a function of the mode of ingestion and the half-life of the drug. Other effects include analgesia, mental clouding, constipation, pupillary constriction, depressed cough reflux, emesis, sweating, and peripheral vasodilation. If the opiate level is sufficiently high, loss of consciousness and respiratory depression can occur. In any instance of decreased level of consciousness where there is a suspicion of opiate overdose, a naloxone challenge should be performed. Because naloxone has a shorter half-life than many opioid agonists, repeated administrations will be necessary to counter the effects of the agonists.

Some of the effects mentioned above (e.g., analgesia, depressed cough reflex, and constipation) can be therapeutic effects of opiates. However, nearly all of these can be severe side effects and/or telltale signs of opiate use. Constipation can be severe, and chronic analgesic use of opiates often requires prescription of stool softeners. A depressed cough reflex can lead to aspiration and pneumonia.

Withdrawal from heroin and other opiates is less dangerous than alcohol withdrawal in terms of mortality but is subjectively very unpleasant for the addict. The difference between physiologic dependence and addiction is perhaps most relevant to opiate drugs but is also very relevant to benzodiazepine abuse. The clinician should note that physiologic signs of tolerance and withdrawal are only two of the required three symptoms necessary to make a substance dependence diagnosis. The other symptoms, which are essentially symptoms of loss of control, compulsive use, and use despite negative consequences, define the behavioral syndrome of addiction. In the case of opiates, it is possible for someone to be physically dependent, and therefore at risk for withdrawal, without being addicted.

The time course of opiate withdrawal varies according to the half-life of the opiate used (Hirsch et al. 1996). For example, heroin withdrawal starts within hours of the last ingestion, peaks over 1–3 days, and resolves within a week. In contrast, methadone withdrawal can take 2 weeks and can be harder to tolerate. Withdrawal symptoms are often divided into early, middle, and late symptoms. Early in the course of withdrawal, anxiety, myalgias, pupillary dilatation, rhinorrhea, and tearing as well as yawning predominate. As the withdrawal continues, sweats, fever, chills, "gooseflesh," insomnia, and muscle and bone pain increase. Finally, vomiting, diarrhea, increased blood pressure, and tachycardia are observed. Of particular importance in the era of naltrexone use for alcohol and opiate addiction is the possibility of inadvertently precipitating opiate withdrawal by giving naltrexone to a person with an unsuspected opiate addiction. Precipitated withdrawal with naltrexone can be very intense and will last about 24 hours (as opposed to 1 hour with naloxone). All patients being considered for naltrexone for alcohol dependence should be thoroughly educated about this phenomenon, given a urine toxicology screen, and potentially given a naloxone test dose.

Treatment for opiate withdrawal involves opiate and nonopiate approaches. Currently, the most frequently used nonopiate drug regimen employs clonidine to decrease the symptoms of withdrawal, because many symptoms result from overactivity of the locus coeruleus and sympathetic nervous system. Treatment with clonidine is superior to placebo, but in the experience of many clinicians and addicts, it is less satisfactory than opiate replacement. It is probably best suited for use in the treatment of patients who have become addicted to oral analgesics and are relatively less dependent.

The treatment of opiate addicts with opiates, for maintenance or withdrawal, requires a special license. Methadone, the long-acting opiate agonist most often prescribed for withdrawal, can be tapered over a 30–180-day withdrawal period. However, relapse is common.

Marijuana and Other Tetrahydrocannabinols

Intoxication with marijuana and other cannabinoids is characterized by slowed reflexes and decreased coordination (Losken et al. 1996; Millman and Beeder 1994). This becomes particularly problematic when people are attempting to operate heavy equipment or drive a motor vehicle. There is currently considerable debate about the medical uses of marijuana, and although federal regulations clearly outlaw its use, some states and municipalities have approved its use for certain medical conditions (Voth and Schwartz 1997).

Chronic use of marijuana can be associated with several problems (Hubbard et al. 1999). Weight gain and the possibility of a mild apathetic dementia have been suggested. Subtle alterations in the immune system have also been described (Klein et al. 1998). Marijuana smoke also places one at risk for the development of lung abnormalities, including cancer. DSM-IV-TR does not include a diagnosis of withdrawal associated with marijuana or other cannabinoids. However, an irritable or anxious mood with tremor, nausea, or perspiration can be associated with the discontinuation of cannabinoids in heavy users (Losken et al. 1996).

Hallucinogens

The two hallucinogens most commonly encountered in clinical practice are lysergic acid diethylamide (LSD) and 3,4-methylenedioxymethamphetamine (MDMA/ecstasy) (Cassidy and Ballard 1994). Both are associated with perceptual distortions rather than with frank hallucinations (Brendel et al. 1996). Patients report the altered perceptions in various ways, but insight that the effect is being caused by a drug is usually maintained (Ungerleider and Pechnick 1994). A diagnosis of drug-induced psychosis is considered for a patient who loses insight into the drug's role in the altered sensory experiences. Such psychoses usually resolve promptly, and the persistence of psychotic symptoms suggests the need to consider alternative diagnoses such as schizophrenia. Although hallucinogens have been suspected of inducing long-term psychiatric syndromes, results of prospective studies are controversial, and no clear long-term adverse sequelae have been documented (Brendel et al. 1996).

Intoxication with hallucinogens is usually characterized by mild signs of autonomic arousal such as tachycardia and pupillary dilatation (Brendel et al. 1996). Keeping the subject in a protective environment and "talking them down" usually is sufficient. MDMA can also cause hypothermia. If ingested in a hot environment, it can lead to dehydration and possibly rhabdomyolysis.

Phencyclidine

PCP intoxication is characterized by an admixture of sedation, lethargy, and agitation (Baldridge and Bessen 1990). Agitation can be of psychotic intensity and characterized by rage attacks and episodes of violent behavior (Brust 1993). Because PCP is stored in fat tissue and released at unpredictable rates, the effects of PCP intoxication can wax and wane over time. Individuals intoxicated with PCP are also very sensitive to noise and therefore should not be "talked down," as is done with hallucinogen-intoxicated patients. They also seem relatively insensitive to pain, a factor that, combined with rage attacks, may lead to acts of violence against self or others. PCP intoxication is also characterized by nystagmus and rigidity (Daghestani and Schnoll 1994).

Drug Testing

The diagnosis of drug intoxication can be made much more confidently when the presence of the drug is confirmed by drug testing. However, what constitutes a toxicity screening varies from institution to institution. It is important for the clinician to know what drugs are tested for when such a screen is ordered and over what period of time a test will remain positive following ingestion of a drug. Typically, screens involve radioimmunoassay or thin-layer chromatography testing for drugs in urine or serum. Many standard radioimmunoassay panels do not detect alcohol, LSD, methadone, meperidine, fentanyl, benzodiazepines, or barbiturates. Thin-layer chromatography, although a more cumbersome procedure and somewhat less reliable, screens for a broader array of drugs.

The period over which tests remain positive varies dramatically from drug to drug. For example, marijuana can often be detected in the urine of chronic users for up to 30 days after discontinuation, whereas cocaine is detectable for less than 2 days in most standard assays. The clinician also must bear in mind the need to obtain samples by direct observation. Clinicians also need to be aware of substances that will give false positive results. For example, a single poppy seed muffin can give a false positive result on some opiate screens.

Medical Complications of Intravenous Drug Administration

Many of the problems that develop in drug abusers are directly attributable to the use of the intravenous route of administration (Kemp et al. 1998). Some of these, such as AIDS, infective endocarditis, hepatitis, renal infections, and skin and soft tissue infections, relate directly to the introduction of pathogens through contaminated needles. Others relate more to the debilitation and malnutrition often seen in these patients. These include pneumonia and tuberculosis (Novick et al. 1997).

Pneumonia, a disorder not necessarily directly linked to substance abuse in the minds of many physicians, is actually one of the most common reasons intravenous drug users are hospitalized. Many factors may contribute, such as poor dental hygiene and aspiration due to suppression of gag and cough reflexes by sedation. Malnutrition and the smoking of cigarettes, marijuana, and/or crack lead to suppression of the immune system. Pneumococcal pneumonia remains the most common form of pneumonia in substance abusers, although *Klebsiella* and *Haemophilus influenzae* strains are also common pathogens. *Pneumocystis carinii* pneumonia occurs most commonly among HIV-infected patients (Novick et al. 1997). Although the initial evaluation for pneumonia (e.g., chest X ray, sputum for Gram's stain and culture, blood cultures, blood gases) might be initiated by the psychiatrist, for definitive evaluation and treatment, the patient needs to be referred to a family practitioner or internist.

In the early 1990s the United States experienced a reversal in what had been a decades-long trend of decreasing prevalence of tuberculosis. The extent to which that increase was attributable to the increased numbers of substance abusers and HIV-infected individuals is not definitely known; multiple other factors were clearly important. All drug users should be screened with a purified protein derivative, and a positive result should prompt more extensive evaluation. Active tuberculosis requires multiple drug therapy, which must be supervised by a specialist.

Infective endocarditis carries a high risk for morbidity and mortality (Novick et al. 1997). The onset of a new murmur in an intravenous drug user who is febrile is suggestive of, but not required for, a diagnosis of endocarditis. Given the unreliability of many intravenous substance abusers as historians and the frequent need to evaluate these patients without access to previous records, the clinician is often in the situation of evaluating a patient with incomplete historical data. The possibility that endocarditis is present should be considered in all intravenous drug abusers who are febrile.

Viral hepatitis is a frequent problem in patients with intravenous drug abuse (Alter and Moyer 1998; Boazhang et al. 1997; Booth 1998; Novick et al. 1997; Steffen and Gutzwiller 1999). The discovery of several types of viral hepatitis over the last 10 years can be somewhat bewildering to the clinician. In brief, the hepatitis A and B viruses have been identified as pathogens for the longest period of time. When it became obvious in the late 1970s that hepatitis A and B did not account for many cases of hepatitis, the search for other viral pathogens intensified. Hepatitis C has now been isolated as the cause of many, but not all, Non-A/Non-B hepatitis cases. Most recently, hepatitis D, an atypical virus that is an obligatory co-infectant with hepatitis B, and hepatitis G, a relatively common independent pathogen, have been isolated. Nearly half of all intravenous drug abusers have a history of hepatitis. The management of the patient with hepatitis C is changing rapidly. Any psychiatrist working with these patients would be advised to consult regularly with gastrointestinal specialists to help the patient understand and comply with treatment and assessment protocols.

The development of skin or soft tissue abscesses is relatively common among intravenous drug abusers and may be accompanied by systemic infection (Novick et al. 1997). Sexually transmitted diseases and AIDS, also common problems among intravenous drug abusers, are covered in Chapter 2.

SUMMARY

In this chapter we attempt to outline some of the more common medical complications that develop during alcohol and drug intoxication or withdrawal. Clinicians often encounter patients in these situations, and it is important for them to be able to recognize such complications and to initiate appropriate evaluation and facilitate needed referrals.

REFERENCES

Allen J, Litten RZ, Lee A: What you need to know: detecting alcohol problems in general medical practice. Singapore Med J 39:38–41, 1998

Alter MJ, Moyer LA: The importance of preventing hepatitis C virus infection among injection drug uses in the United States. J Acquir Immune Defic Syndr 18:S6–S10, 1998

American Psychiatric Association: Diagnostic and Statistical Manual of Mental Disorders, 4th Edition Text Revision. Washington, DC, American Psychiatric Association, 2000

Amurawaiye EO, Brown RA: Acute pancreatitis: 30 years' experience at a teaching hospital. Can J Surg 34:137–143, 1991

Baldridge EB, Bessen HA: Phencyclidine. Emerg Med Clin North Am 8:541–550, 1990

Baozhang T, Kaining Z, Jinxing K, et al: Infection with human immunodeficiency virus and hepatitis viruses in Chinese drug addicts. Epidemiol Infect 119:343–347, 1997

Beresford TP: Predictive factors for alcohol relapse in the selection of alcohol-dependent persons for hepatic transplant. Liver Transpl 3:280–291, 1997

Boghdadi MS, Henning RJ: Cocaine: pathophysiology and clinical toxicology. Heart Lung 26:466–483, 1997

Booth JC: Chronic hepatitis C: the virus, its discovery and the natural history of the disease. J Viral Hepat 5:213–222, 1998

Brendel D, West H, Hyman SE: Hallucinogens and phencyclidine, in Source Book of Substance Abuse and Addiction. Edited by Friedman LS, Fleming NF, Roberts DH, et al. Baltimore, MD, Williams & Wilkins, 1996, pp 217–229

Brust JC: Other agents: phencyclidine, marijuana, hallucinaogens, inhalants, and anticholinergics. Neurol Clin 11:555–561, 1993

Cassidy GC, Ballard G: Psychiatric sequele of MDMA (ecstasy) and related drugs. International Journal of Psychiatry in Medicine 11:132–133, 1994

Cook CA, Booth BM, Blow FC, et al: Alcoholism treatment, severity of alcohol-related medical complications, and health services utilization. J Ment Health Adm 19:31–40, 1992

Crabb DW: Pathogenesis of alcoholic liver disease: newer mechanisms of injury. Keio J Med 48:184–188, 1999

Daghestani AN, Schnoll SH: Phencyclidine, in The American Psychiatric Press Textbook of Substance Abuse Treatment. Edited by Galanter M and Kleber HD. Washington, DC, American Psychiatric Press, 1994, pp 149–156

D'Amour ML, Butterworth RF: Pathogenesis of alcohol peripheral neuropathy: direct effect of ethanol or nutritional deficit? Metab Brain Dis 9:133–142, 1994

Dawson DA: Drinking as a risk factor for sustained smoking. Drug and Alcohol Dependence 59: 235–249, 2000

Diamond I, Messing RO: Neurologic effects of alcoholism. West J Med 161:279–287, 1994

Erstad BL, Cotugno CL: Management of alcohol withdrawal. Am J Health Syst Pharm 52: 697–709, 1995

Fenster F: Alcohol and disorders of the gastrointestinal system, in Alcoholism: Development, Consequences, and Interventions. Edited by Estes NJ, Heinemann ME. St. Louis, MO, Mosby, 1986, pp 145–152

Fernando OV, Grimsley EW: Prevalence of folate deficiency and macrocytosis in patients with and without alcohol-related illnesses. South Med J 91:721–725, 1998

Galanter M, Kleber HD (eds): The American Psychiatric Press Textbook of Substance Abuse Treatment. Washington, DC, American Psychiatric Press, 1994

Gallant D: Alcohol, in The American Psychiatric Press Textbook of Substance Abuse Treatment. Edited by Galanter M, Kleber HD. Washington, DC, American Psychiatric Press, 1994, pp 67–89

Gawin FH: Cocaine addiction: psychology and neurophysiology. Science 251:1580–1586, 1991

Gawin FH, Khalsa-Denison ME: Is craving mood-driven or self-propelled? Sensitization and "street" stimulant addiction. NIDA Res Monogr 163:224–250, 1996

Harris D, Brunt P: Prognosis of alcoholic liver disease: 100 years on and the need for international standards and guidelines. Alcohol Alcohol 30:591–600, 1995

Hillman RS: Hematologic disorders of alcoholism, in Alcoholism: Development, Consequences, and Interventions. Edited by Estes NJ, Heinemann ME. St. Louis, MO, Mosby, 1986, pp 176–183

Hirsch D, Paley JE, Renner Jr JA: Opiates, in Source Book of Substance Abuse and Addiction. Edited by Friedman LS, Fleming NF, Roberts DH, et al. Baltimore, MD, Williams & Wilkins, 1996, pp 189–202

Hubbard JR, Franco SE, Onaivi ES: Marijuana: medical implications. Am Fam Physician 60:2583–2588, 2593, 1999

Isla AM: Chronic pancreatitis. Hosp Med 61:386–389, 2000

Jones AW: Aspects of in-vivo pharmacokinetics of ethanol. Alcohol Clin Exp Res 24:400–402, 2000

Keeffe EB: Assessment of the alcoholic patient for liver transplantation: comorbidity, outcome, and recidivism. Liver Transpl Surg 2:12–20, 1996

Kemp R, Miller J, Lungley S, et al: Injecting behaviours and prevalence of hepatitis B, C and D markers in New Zealand injecting drug user populations. N Z Med J 111:50–53, 1998

Kerfoot BP, Sakoulas G, Hyman SE: Cocaine, in Source Book of Substance Abuse and Addiction. Edited by Friedman LS, Fleming NF, Roberts DH, et al. Baltimore, MD, Williams & Wilkins, 1996, pp 157–178

Klein TW, Friedman H, Specter S: Marijuana, immunity, and infection. J Neuroimmunol 83:102–115, 1998

Kushner SF: Substance abuse and neurological disorders, in Dual Diagnosis in Substance Abuse. Edited by Gold MS, Slaby AE. New York, Marcel Dekker, 1991, pp 75–103

Li TK, Beard JD, Orr WE, et al: Variation in ethanol pharmacokinetics and perceived gender and ethnic differences in alcohol elimination. Alcohol Clin Exp Res 24:415–416, 2000

Lieber CS: Hepatic and other medial disorders of alcoholism: from pathogenesis to treatment. J Stud Alcohol 59:9–25, 1998

Lieber CS: Alcoholic liver disease: new insights in pathogenesis lead to new treatments. J Hepatol 32:113–128, 2000

Lieber CS, Abittan CS: Pharmacology and metabolism of alcohol, including its metabolic effects and interactions with other drugs. Clin Dermatol 17:365–379, 1999

Losken A, Maviglia S, Friedman LS: Marijuana, in Source Book of Substance Abuse and Addiction. Edited by Friedman LS, Fleming NF, Roberts DH, et al. Baltimore, MD, Williams & Wilkins, 1996, pp 179–187

Lucey MR: Liver transplantation for the alcoholic patient. Gastroenterol Clin North Am 22:243–256, 1993

MacDonald J, Twardon EM, Shafer HJ: Alcohol, in Source Book of Substance Abuse and Addiction. Edited by Friedman LS, Fleming NF, Roberts DH, et al. Baltimore, MD, Williams & Wilkins, 1996, pp 109–137

Maisch B: Alcohol and the heart. Herz 21:207–212, 1996

Masand PS, Sousou AJ, Gupta S, et al: Irritable bowel syndrome (IBS) and alcohol abuse or dependence. Am J Drug Alcohol Abuse 24:513–521, 1998

McIlvain HE, Bobo JK, Leed-Kelly A, et al: Practical steps to smoking cessation for recovering alcoholics. Am Fam Physician 57:1869–1876, 1998

Millman RB, Beeder AB: Cannabis. in The American Psychiatric Press Textbook of Substance Abuse Treatment. Edited by Galanter M, Kleber HD. Washington, DC, American Psychiatric Press, 1994, pp 91–109

Mumenthaler MS, Taylor JL, O'Hara R, et al: Gender differences in moderate drinking effects. Alcohol Res Health 23:55–64, 1999

Munoz A, Katerndahl DA: Diagnosis and management of acute pancreatitis. Am Fam Physician 62:164–174, 2000

Novick DM, Haverkos HW, Teller DW: The medically ill substance abuser, in Substance Abuse: A Comprehensive Textbook, 3rd Edition. Edited by Lowinson JH, Ruiz P, Millman RB, et al. Baltimore, MD, Williams & Wilkins, 1997, pp 534–563

O'Malley SS, Gawin FH: Abstinence symptomatology and neuropsychological impairment in chronic cocaine abusers. NIDA Res Monogr 101:179–190, 1990

Oslin D, Atkinson RM, Smith DM, et al: Alcohol-related dementia: proposed clinical criteria. Int J Geriatr Psychiatry 13:203–212, 1998

Ozdemir V, Bremner KE, Naranjo CA: Treatment of alcohol withdrawal syndrome. Ann Med 26:101–105, 1994

Petitti DB, Sidney S, Quesenberry C, et al: Stroke and cocaine or amphetamine use. Epidemiology 9:596–600, 1998

Pitchumoni CS: Chronic pancreatitis: a historical and clinical sketch of the pancreas and pancreatitis. Gastroenterologist 6:24–33, 1998

Portenoy RK, Payne R: Acute and chronic pain, in Substance Abuse: A Comprehensive Textbook, 3rd Edition. Edited by Lowinson JH, Ruiz P, Millman RB, et al. Baltimore, MD, Williams & Wilkins, 1997, pp 563–589

Rubin E, Urbano-Marquez A: Alcoholic cardiomyopathy. Alcohol Clin Exp Res 18:111–114, 1994

Schenker S, Bay MK: Medical problems associated with alcoholism. Adv Intern Med 43:27–78, 1998

Severinghaus J, Kinney J: Medical management, in Clinical Manual of Substance Abuse, 2nd Edition. Edited by Kinney J. St. Louis, MO, Mosby-Year Book, 1996, pp 99–128

Smith JW: Alcohol and disorders of the heart and skeletal muscles, in Alcoholism: Development, Consequences, and Interventions. Edited by Estes NJ, Heinemann ME. St. Louis, MO, Mosby, 1986a, pp 184–192

Smith JW: Neurologic disorders in alcoholism, in Alcoholism: Development, Consequences, and Interventions. Edited by Estes NJ, Heinemann ME. St. Louis, MO, Mosby, 1986b, pp 153–175

Steffen T, Gutzwiller F: Hepatitis B and C in intravenous drug abusers in Switzerland. Schweiz Rundsch Med Prax 88:1937–1944, 1999

Ungerleider JT, Pechnick RN: Hallucinogens, in The American Psychiatric Press Textbook of Substance Abuse Treatment. Edited by Galanter M, Kleber HD. Washington, DC, American Psychiatric Press, 1994, pp 141–147

Voth EA, Schwartz RH: Medicinal applications of delta-9-tetrahydrocannabinol and marijuana. Ann Intern Med 126:791–798, 1997

Worthington-Roberts B: Alcoholism and malnutrition, in Alcoholism: Development, Consequences, and Interventions. Edited by Estes NJ, Heinemann ME. St. Louis, MO, Mosby, 1986, pp 110–144

Zullino D, Beeson J, Schnyder C: Stage of change of cigarette smoking in alcohol-dependent patients. Eur Addict Res 6:84–90, 2000

Index

*Page numbers printed in **boldface** type refer to tables.*